eat

YOUR WAY TO

HAPPINESS

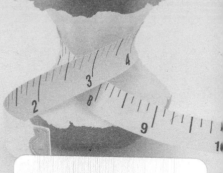

eat

YOUR WAY TO

HAPPINESS

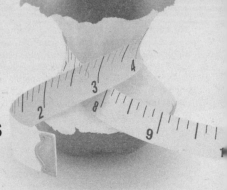

DROP THE POUNDS

BOOST YOUR MOOD

CONQUER YOUR CRAVINGS

Elizabeth Somer, M.A., R.D.

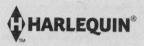

HARLEQUIN®

EAT YOUR WAY TO HAPPINESS
ISBN-13: 978-0-373-89268-6

© 2009 by Elizabeth Somer

Recycling programs for this product may not exist in your area.

The nutritional and health advice presented in this book is based on an in-depth review of the current scientific literature. It is intended only as an informative resource guide to help you make informed decisions; it is not meant to replace the advice of a physician or to serve as a guide to self-treatment. Always seek competent medical help for any health condition or if there is any question about the appropriateness of a procedure or health recommendation.

A full list of references used in the writing of this book can be found at www.ElizabethSomer.com.

www.Harlequin.com

Printed in U.S.A.

To all the kind and happy people in my life.

The Dalai Lama says that the purpose of life is to seek happiness. Happy people automatically are more generous and less self-focused, which means they naturally enrich the lives of all those around them. The world is a kinder, safer, more loving and joyful place because they are in it.

CONTENTS

Secret 2: Follow the 1-2-3 Rule

Secret 3: Choose Quality Carbs

Secret 4: Adopt the 6% Solution

Secret 5: Sprinkle It with Super Mood Foods

Secret 6: Embrace the Good Fat

Secret 7: Get Smart with Supplements

Secret 8: Choose the Right Thirst Quenchers

Secret 9: Indulge in the Right Vices

Secret 10: Eat Right at Night

Secret 11: The One Habit You Must Embrace to Be Happy, Fit and Healthy

ACKNOWLEDGMENTS

A heartfelt thank-you to all the friends, family members, coworkers, clients, students and acquaintances who made this book possible. First, thank you to David Smith, the best agent in the world, and a dear friend. Thank you to my editor, Deborah Brody, who has seen me through many projects and who I still can sidetrack from editing issues or title ponderings with the mere mention of a bike ride. Thank you to all the people who so graciously shared their stories, accomplishments and solutions—you will read all their successes in the pages that follow. I am indebted to the researchers whose dedication and hard work provide the basis for the accurate and reliable information on which I have based my entire career. A huge "thank you" to my two perfect kids, Lauren and Will, for just being in my life and filling me with joy, pride and love.

INTRODUCTION

Blissfully thin. Take a moment to imagine what that would be like—to be joyously happy, fit, trim and sexy.

What would it feel like to wake up each morning after a deep and restful sleep, filled with energy, enthusiasm and anticipation of another wonderful day ahead of you? To have all the energy and mental sharpness to tackle any task that came your way, to thoroughly enjoy your job, family, friends and activities? To be filled to the brim every day with gratitude and hope, excitement and inner peace? To be calm, relaxed, at peace with yourself, your world, your future and your life?

What would it feel like to be lean, fit, confident and strong? To slip easily into a little black dress or the jeans you wore in high school? To have the energy and strength to bound up a flight of stairs, work in the yard all day with energy to spare, enjoy long hikes with the family or take up tennis? To feel comfortable in your own skin and to feel proud of yourself and desirable to others?

Accept that all of that is possible.

The Promise

No diet, book or teacher can guarantee bliss or a perfect figure for the rest of your life, just as no one can guarantee you will live disease-free until you die peacefully in your sleep at age 110. But I can promise that if you follow the secrets laid out in this book, you will stack the deck in favor of being blissfully fit. I also promise that if you follow my advice in the pages that follow you will feel the best you have felt in a long time, if ever, and will be thinner and fitter than you've ever been in your adult life.

How do I know that? I have been researching the link between diet and mood for decades. That research led me to write *Food & Mood,* which came out in its first edition in 1995. Since then, people have been sharing their stories with me of how that book changed their lives.

People have told me they followed my diet advice and found a new lease on life. Young, old, kids, teenagers, men and women all got happier, leaner, smarter or less stressed. Their energy improved. Their memories returned. They slept better, reacted faster, handled stress better. Menopausal women told me their hot flashes disappeared, men told me they no longer fell asleep in the recliner every night. Many times their depression lifted, or they were able to discontinue, or at least reduce, their medications. Often PMS symptoms vanished, or they no longer battled the Winter

Blues. They were enthusiastic about life and looked forward to the future. I wish I had a dollar for every time someone told me, "I never knew I could feel this good!"

Michelle, a producer for NBC's *Today* show, is a perfect example. When she was 12 years old, she was hit head-on by a car. "The car continued to drive with me on the windshield, and I eventually fell to the street and suffered a second blow to my head," she told me. She was left with a traumatic brain injury, as well as back and neck problems. As a result of the brain injury, she forgot how to read and do any type of math. "Even something as simple as subtracting the number 6 from 10 was difficult for me in those early years. I suffered extreme anxiety and fell into a depression as well."

Slowly Michelle regained her life, her mind and her mood:

"Good nutrition and health played a *huge* role in my recovery. It was Elizabeth's advice about how to eat to improve my mood that helped me understand the power of foods and the effects of my eating habits on my brain and body. I gave up sugar and refined carbs and added in all the good stuff, especially depression-fighting foods she recommended, like salmon and berries. I made a full recovery and have accomplished more than anyone ever thought I would.

I graduated from college with honors, served as a White House intern and now work for NBC's #1 morning show. I can't tell you how important eating well was in my recovery. It gave me the energy, determination and health I needed to battle my injuries. *Food & Mood* was my bible. I'm so grateful that something inspired me to pull that book off my mom's bookshelf. I can't imagine where I'd be today without it."

You Are Exactly What You Eat

You've heard the old adage "You are what you eat." Most of us realize the truth of that statement when it comes to our physical health. We know if we drink soda instead of calcium-rich milk that somewhere down the road we are likely to end up with bone loss and osteoporosis. We know that a diet loaded with greasy fast foods will cause heart disease, at least someday. Maybe you supplement with a few extra antioxidants in hopes of slowing the aging process.

I am in full support of getting enough calcium for your bones, cutting back on the saturated fat to protect arteries and getting all the antioxidants you can to slow aging. However, it takes months, years, even decades for a bad diet to show up as a physical problem, while the link between your diet and your mood is much more immediate.

Literally, what you eat or don't eat for breakfast will affect how well you feel, how much energy you have and how clearly you think by midafternoon. What you have for lunch may well determine how sharp you are midafternoon or set the stage for whether you battle cravings at night for buttery popcorn or gallons of ice cream. It also might affect how well you sleep that night, which then affects how alert and energetic you are the next day.

Janet, an editor and actor in Southern California, says,

> "When I eat the right breakfast, keep my lunch and dinner light, balance protein with quality carbs and definitely cut way back on sweets, I have tons of energy, sleep better and think more clearly. Also, I noticed that when I overindulge in 'junk' eating, I become oversensitive and 'weepy,' which is definitely not me. What a wake-up call for how food can affect me emotionally!"

Of course, your food choices today affect your long-term mood and mind, too. What you eat and how you supplement today will have a huge impact on whether you are depressed, develop dementia or Alzheimer's, or lose your independence in later years. In fact, the better care you take of yourself today, the more likely you will live disease-free, sharp-as-a-tack and independent into your nineties or beyond. As one researcher put it, "the older you get, the healthier you've been."

It Just Makes Sense

Every atom, every molecule, every cell, tissue, organ and system in your body is made up of the ingredients in the foods you eat, the water you drink and the air you breathe. Cell membranes are made up of fats and proteins from foods like the salmon or nuts you had for lunch. The iron in your red blood cells that carries oxygen to your brain and tissues comes from something as simple as the black beans in a burrito. The energy your brain uses to relay messages comes from the carbs in a bowl of cereal at breakfast, and the B vitamins that convert those carbs into cell energy came from the milk you poured over the cereal. So it just makes sense that you literally are exactly what you choose to eat.

There are 40+ nutrients and more than 12,000 phytonutrients in foods that your body and brain can't make by itself but require to function in tip-top shape. The amount and balance of those thousands of nutrients determines whether you are happy or sad, smart or forgetful, energetic or lethargic, healthy or diseased, living vibrantly or dragging through the day.

Every sprig of broccoli, every leaf of spinach, every bite of tuna or egg or potato is converted into the living organism your friends call *you*. Give your body the right mix of the right nutrients at the right time, and your body hums along like a well-oiled, highly tuned, perfectly timed machine. Feed it junk, and it's no surprise you feel horrible, gain weight and are likely to age before your time.

You Aren't the First Human to Need Vitamin C

You know deep down in your heart that eating junk is bad for you. Sure, it might feel good to curl up on the couch with a half-gallon of ice cream on a lonely Friday night. But too many of those temporary indulgences always backfires. Always. Eat crap and that's how you will feel: physically, emotionally and mentally...today, tomorrow and years down the road.

Just as junk brings you down, eating the right mood-boosting foods—the type of foods that the human body evolved to need and thrive on—and including those foods in the right amounts at the right times can be one of life's most permanent uplifting experiences. Food really can be the way to a *natural high!* When you set aside the immediate gratification of eating a gooey, sticky, greasy, sweet glob of junk, and instead feed your body the foods on which it thrives—foods known to improve mood and slim waistlines—you will be amazed how good you feel, how much energy you have, how smart you are, how the pounds just melt away and how the mood pendulum swings from guilt and depression to pride and joy. I know because I've researched this topic for almost 20 years and have seen the results firsthand over and over and over again.

Just Take a Pill?

Oh sure, you can take medications to treat depression, anxiety and other emotional problems. In fact, medications like selective serotonin reuptake inhibitors (i.e., Prozac) are the number one treatment option for depression. I'm not against that solution when all else fails. The problem is most mood-altering medications come with a slew of side effects. Many antidepressants, for example, cause weight gain, make you drowsy and lethargic, ruin your sex drive, slow metabolism or mess with your blood sugar.

I can understand why people would be willing to make the trade and put up with those side effects just to feel good again. However, medication is not always the holy grail for depression.

You should always seek medical help if the blues last more than a month or are accompanied by other symptoms. In all cases, however, even if you choose to begin with medication or therapy, diet always will help. A change in what and how you eat has benefits that are more immediate than those often experienced with drugs, with improvements sometimes noted within as little as one to three weeks. What you eat can be the ultimate *natural high,* since it comes with no side effects except a lowered risk for all diseases and an increased chance of living longer, smarter, healthier and leaner. In many cases, a change in diet is all you need to feel better and drop pounds.

Following the guidelines in this book will help speed your return to happiness with or without medication. The guidelines are the natural-high solution to lifelong joy and a fit figure. The more closely you follow the secrets and advice in this book, the faster and more dramatic will be your results. But any change, even small ones, will help turn the emotional tide.

The Latest and the Best

We've come a long way in the past decade or two when it comes to understanding how food affects mood, mind and energy. This book is a culmination of extensive research and experience, coupled with some amazing breakthroughs and new foods that speed the process of feeling your best by eating right. The following pages are filled with people's stories of how making a few changes in what and when they ate turned out to be the ticket to joy and a sleeker figure.

In the next few chapters, you'll learn the top 10 diet secrets to happiness, distilled from decades of research and personal experience. You'll learn simple ways to tweak your diet that will have profound effects on how good you feel, how consistent your mood is, how sharp your mind is, and how energetic you can be, while you lose weight and regain your health.

Self-Assessment: Are You Blue?

Are you a bit iffy as to whether your mood is normal or teeters on depression? This quiz is by no means meant to replace a physician's diagnosis, but it might help you determine if you need to make an appointment. The more "yes" answers, the more likely you are to be bluer than normal.

		No	Yes
1.	I feel tired or even lethargic several times during the weekday	○	○
2.	I am unmotivated most of the day	○	○
3.	Seldom does anything bring me true joy	○	○
4.	I am sad most of the day	○	○
5.	I get teary over even unimportant things	○	○
6.	Several times a week, I feel hopeless or worthless	○	○
7.	I frequently have trouble concentrating	○	○
8.	People have commented on my sad or anxious mood	○	○
9.	I sleep poorly more than once a week	○	○
10.	I frequently turn to food, especially sweets, or alcohol, in the hopes of feeling better	○	○
11.	I have lost interest in activities, people, events that I once enjoyed	○	○
12.	I've lost interest in sex	○	○
13.	Sometimes I think that putting an end to my life would be the easiest option	○	○
14.	I think about death a lot	○	○

Which Comes First: The Mood or the Food?

How you feel and your weight are a chicken-and-egg match made in either heaven or hell. If you are happy (and I mean really happy, not just on-the-surface, pretend happy), you also are most likely to be leaner.

As people lose weight, their moods improve, or vica versa—as their moods improve, they lose weight. As their moods improve and they lose weight, they cut their risk in half for a whole host of ills, from heart disease to diabetes, in part because they are more motivated to take good care of themselves. But the link goes further than that. Boost their happiness quotient and they lower stress hormones, such as cortisol, and the inflammatory processes associated with disease. Lower stress means people sleep better, think more clearly and have more energy, which are all factors that help them lose weight and stay happy.

Additionally, people with sunny outlooks are more likely to choose healthy foods, which in turn fuel their good moods. They are less likely to get sick, they recover more quickly if they do get sick, they live longer—more than 7 and possibly up to 10 years longer—and they are healthier in those extra years than are people who are either depressed and/or overweight. It works in reverse, too. People who choose foods known to improve mood find it easier to lose weight, cope with stress and sleep better.

The opposite also is true. When people are over-weight, they are most likely to feel sluggish, not sexy, tired and depressed. They turn to food—typically the wrong ones!—to soothe the gloom, which adds more weight and stress, disrupts their sleep and drops their mood even further. Poor sleep habits, in turn, increase the risk for being overweight...some studies found by up to 70%. It's no surprise that people who are sad or downright depressed are twice as likely to be overweight, and people who are overweight are twice as likely to become depressed and anxious and suffer other mental health problems. For example, a potbelly at age 50 more than triples the risk for dementia by the time someone hits the senior years! Those people also are at highest risk for atherosclerosis, diabetes, high blood pressure, memory loss, osteoporosis and dementia.

The trick here is to make that chicken-and-egg scenario work in your favor. You can jump in anywhere in the cycle, put on the brakes and reverse the process, spiraling up out of depression and weight gain and into the sunshine of happiness and a fit figure. Adopt some of the secrets in this book, guaranteed to improve your outlook on life and slim your waistline, and you will feel better, more hopeful, happier and lighter. The better and more energetic you feel, the more motivated you will be to stick with it, the more weight you'll lose, the better you'll feel, and so on.

I've seen it happen for so many people over the years, and I know it can work for you, too.

Janet knows firsthand how changing your diet can turn your life around:

"I was a breakfast avoider for many years, especially when I worked full-time. Or I'd chow down on coffee, muffins and, in my earlier years, cigarettes. Could I have been more unhealthy if I tried?! Then, if that was not enough, lunch was always something from the fast-food places on campus—Mexican, Chinese or the deli. I was so used to dragging myself to work then dragging myself home for a nap, I didn't even realize how bad I felt. Everyone warned me that once I stopped working full-time I would gain tons of weight, but they were wrong. I took the time off from working as an opportunity to care for myself. I changed most of those unhealthy habits, started eating a sane breakfast and a light lunch, and included more of the feel-good foods that I knew would help me think better and energize my day. You know what happened? I lost 30 pounds! My stress levels went down. I felt so good that I got up the nerve to dive into my passion, which always has been acting. Today I have more energy and am a much happier human being, and it all started by making a few simple adjustments to my diet!"

The Happy Diet

We not only are what we eat, but certain foods tweak our brain chemistry and help us stay happy, energized and even calm. One example of how what we eat affects how we feel is the relationship between carbs and serotonin. It is no coincidence that we turn to carbs, from pasta to cookies, when we are in a foul frame of mind. Carb-rich foods stimulate the release of a brain chemical called serotonin that regulates appetite, mood and sleep. It makes perfect sense that we crave carbs when we are feeling blue, since these are the very foods that raise serotonin levels and lift our spirits.

Sweets raise levels of another group of brain chemicals called the endorphins. These are the feel-good brain chemicals associated with a runner's high. Chocolate boosts levels of brain chemicals, like phenylethylamine and anandamide, that give us a euphoric or "in love" feeling. The fats in fish alter brain chemistry in favor of being happier and smarter, while the bad fats in meat clog blood vessels in the brain, which muddles thinking and mood.

Mood also affects the foods we eat (anyone who has soothed their anger with a bag of chips or calmed their nerves with a Long Island Iced Tea can relate to that!). For example, stress raises brain levels of another brain chemical called neuropeptide Y (NPY). This brain chemical turns on our appetites for carbs. We overeat and gain weight, which puts us in a funk that adds further stress to our lives, and the cycle goes round and round. Many of those neurotransmitters control both our mood and our cravings, and, like the proverbial chicken and egg, much of what we eat, in turn, turns on and off those neurotransmitters.

How important your diet is to your mood really crystallized for me when I received a phone call from a reporter in Cincinnati. He had called to interview me on the topic of food and mood. "They call me the office curmudgeon. Can you help me?" he asked. He sent me a three-day example of his diet, which immediately explained why he had transformed from an easygoing guy to a grump. First, the only food to grace his lips before noon was a chain of coffees. A light lunch, more coffee, then a huge evening meal just before bedtime was his normal routine. On weekends, he cut back on coffee, which explained why he battled headaches from Saturday to Monday morning (caffeine withdrawal usually includes a whopper of a headache). He was a living example of how to eat to mess up your mood.

After reviewing the reporter's diet, I asked him to make a few changes, such as eating breakfast, including a few super mood foods in his daily menu, cutting back on caffeine and sugar and spreading his food intake more evenly throughout the day. Within no time, his reputation as a curmudgeon had fallen by the wayside. He was more agreeable, enjoyed his job more, no longer battled headaches on the weekends and felt years younger. Granted, healthy foods are not always the cure for clinical depression or other major mood disorders, but following the secrets and advice in this book will always help and is often all it takes to get your mojo back!

You Must Fight for Happiness

Maybe you have tried dieting before. Lost weight, regained it. Lost it again, felt miserable, regained it. If you are a bit gun-shy when it comes to another diet, let me soothe your fears. The eating style I've laid out in this book works, and it doesn't work because it makes you miserable and forces you to live on packaged foods or follow some weird food-combining diet that is more of an eighth-grade science experiment than a gourmet meal. The advice in this book is a get-real approach that combines common sense with the latest research and decades of experience.

People lose weight every day. The trick is to maintain the weight loss and to watch your mood rise as the number on the scale drops. You want the joy and the figure to last. That's what this book is all about.

I promise you *it is not only possible to feel good while dieting, it is absolutely essential to long-term success!* It's a whole lot easier to drop pounds and make changes if you are happy, motivated, energetic and empowered. Your body will drop weight faster when you've had a good night's sleep, are able to cope with stress and can think straight. In short, you must feed your brain while you are trimming your waistline. Luckily, I can tell you just how to do that.

The Catch

Before I get to the details, let's get one thing straight right from the start: no one is effortlessly blessed with happiness and thinness. No one aimlessly wanders through life lean and gleeful. People over the age of 25 who say they can eat whatever they want and never exercise, yet stay skinny and joyful, are lying.

Anyone who is blissfully happy and fit works at it. They get real. They take full responsibility and they take action. They work at it every single day, sometimes at every single meal. They organize, prepare and regroup constantly. They plan ahead, make trade-offs, reward their efforts, occasionally keep records of what and how much they eat and monitor their progress. They stock their kitchens to accommodate healthy eating, they surround themselves with people who support their efforts and they practice thinking like a thin person. They push the self-defeating, negative thoughts out of their heads and replace them with positive, affirming thoughts. They nip in the bud each and every slip that might lead them in the direction toward weight gain and depression. Everyone who is fit and happy has earned it!

Not only does taking charge of your health, life, mood and waistline bring you more happiness than you ever thought possible, as well as allow you to finally get a handle on your weight, but it also is the ticket for ongoing success. A study at the University of Missouri investigated long-term happiness by following students who made intentional changes in their lives to be successful, like joining a club. They compared those "take-charge" students with other students who also had positive experiences that just happened to them, like receiving a scholarship. All the students felt happier at first, but only the ones who had made the effort to deliberately seek happiness stayed that way long-term. You must work to reap the rewards. The more effort you put in, the greater the rewards and the better you'll feel—for the rest of your life.

There's even more good news. I know most people don't like to change habits, diet or make the effort to exercise. Wouldn't it be great if you could just watch TV and get thin and happy? Sorry. Ain't going to happen. You have to put in the effort, but what happy, skinny people find is that the longer you stick with the program, the easier it gets. The longer you follow the secrets in this book, the more likely the changes will become habit.

Self-Assessment:
Do You Eat Like a Happy, Fit Person?

Be completely honest. Do you skip meals sometimes? Snack from the vending machine at work? Occasionally dine from the drive-through? Do you drink soda? Snack on chips? Are you eating to fuel a good mood or depression? Let's get brutally honest. Now is the time to really take a look at what you're eating.

Answer the questions (honestly!) then tally your score to see how you rate and what is working for you and what isn't. Rank your answers 0 to 2 (0 = never, 1 = sometimes, 2 = always).

1. Every day I eat at least eight servings of colorful fruits and/or vegetables (potatoes, fries and iceberg lettuce don't count). _____

2. Every day I eat at least two dark green vegetables such as romaine lettuce, spinach and broccoli. _____

3. Every day I eat at least one dark orange fruit or vegetable, such as carrots, apricots, sweet potatoes or cantaloupe. _____

4. At least five times a week, I eat one or more of the following: nuts, soy, legumes, tart cherries, berries or wheat germ. _____

5. Every day I include in my diet at least one serving of citrus fruit. _____

6. I eat primarily whole grains, including 100% whole-grain breads, cereals, pastas and crackers. _____

7. I average three servings daily of nonfat milk, milk products and/or calcium-fortified soy milk/cheese or OJ. _____

8. I include salmon or other fatty fish in my diet at least twice a week or make sure I get at least 200 milligrams of the omega-3 fat DHA in my daily diet. _____

9. I am careful about my fat intake and only use healthy fats, such as olive oil or oils from nuts. _____

10. I read labels and choose foods with little or no added sugar. I also eat few desserts and always keep the serving size small. _____

11. I limit intake of processed, convenience and fast foods. _____

12. I eat breakfast every day. _____

13. I eat minimeals and snacks throughout the day so that no more than four hours goes by between meals. _____

14. I drink at least eight glasses of water every day. _____

15. If I drink coffee or caffeinated beverages, I do so in moderation (i.e., no more than 24 ounces a day). _____

16. At restaurants, I order low-fat, healthy foods like salads, steamed vegetables, grilled chicken or fish and fresh fruit. I also watch portion sizes. _____

17. I drink alcohol in moderation or not at all (i.e., one drink or less/day). _____

18. I limit my vices to small amounts of red wine, dark chocolate and/or tea a few times a week. _____

19. I take a moderate-dose multiple vitamin and mineral supplement. _____

20. I exercise for at least 30 minutes every day and up to an hour or more three or more days every week. _____

Score:

35 to 40 Outstanding. Your diet borders on perfection. You should be blissfully happy and fit. If not, recheck to make sure you are being completely honest, especially about portion sizes and activity level.

29 to 34 Good job. You are well on your way to being happy and lean. Stick with your current habits, but tweak your eating style to raise those scores lower than 2.

20 to 28 Average. You fit right in with most people, which means there are some changes to be made ASAP. Identify three or four 0 and

1 scores that you want to boost into the 1 to 2 range. When you've successfully accomplished this, tackle two or three more.

0 to 19 Needs serious improvement. Time to start taking your health a whole lot more seriously if you really want to be happier, healthier and leaner. Set a goal to gradually improve your score by three points every month until your score is above 19.

You Deserve the Best

You deserve to feel and look your best. You deserve respect and to feel great. You must believe you are worth it or you'll undermine every attempt you make to re-create yourself, your health, your mood, your weight and your life. You'll only get there if you make the decision and take the responsibility to make it happen. The steps are simple:

- First, believe you deserve it.
- Second, decide you want it.
- Third, get started.
- Fourth, keep at it.

That's what Mary, a retired housewife in Austin, Texas, found. Mary was at least 75 pounds overweight. She wanted desperately to lose the weight yet denied she ate too much. She told me her diet consisted of vegetables, salads, grilled chicken breast and an occasional glass of wine. Mary was lying. Maybe not intentionally, but no one gets that overweight eating broccoli! Mary was in such denial that I finally decided to spend the day with her. The results were anything but surprising.

Mary's kitchen was a telltale sign that more than vegetables were in her diet. Her fridge and cupboards were stocked with foods that would ruin even Pollyanna's Little-Miss-Sunshine mood, including butter, sour cream, whole milk, a variety of cheeses, ice cream, Marie Callendar frozen entrees, store-bought muffins and bottles of alfredo sauce. Her cup of coffee in the morning was more half & half than brew. She tossed the remains of our breakfast in her mouth as she loaded the dishwasher, nibbled on organic trail mix all morning while we talked and then ordered the same salad as I did at the restaurant—only she asked for it with dressing, croutons and cheese, while mine had dressing on the side and neither of the other two.

We spent the entire day on our butts, never once doing any type of physical activity. "I'm having trouble with my hip," she told me, which was her excuse to not exercise. Although dinner was roasted vegetables and chicken breast, the veggies were tossed with almost 600 calories worth of olive oil and the chicken was stuffed with greasy cheese. By the end of the day, Mary had consumed almost 3,000 calories, but she had expended only about 300 calories in the minimal walking we did around the house and from the car to the restaurant. Her 5'5" frame had no other choice than to pocket the extra calories as fat.

Mary's first step in turning around her mood and her figure was to get brutally honest with herself (with a little help from me). Yes, she really wanted to lose the weight; she wasn't just giving lip service to that wish. She agreed to toss the excuses, along with the butter and full-fat dressings, and to pick up a food journal. She kept a detailed record for one week of everything she ate and drank. That record was a blaring wake-up call on the habits she needed to fix. From there, we set to work tweaking her diet to fit the 10 tried-and-true secrets to happiness and a leaner body outlined in this book, which include

1. Focus on real food, not processed junk.
2. Follow the 1-2-3 Rule at breakfast.
3. Choose quality carbs and toss the refined stuff.
4. Use the 6% solution to rein in a sweet tooth.
5. Sprinkle the diet every day with a few super mood foods.
6. Include more mood-boosting fats.
7. Accent the positive by taking the right supplements.
8. Include a few of the right vices in the weekly diet.
9. Get smart about which beverages—and how much—to drink.
10. End the day with the right meal.

The last secret—number 11—is really no secret at all. Mary had to exercise if she was really serious about feeling and looking her best. You do, too. Any diet that tells you otherwise is a con job. Almost everyone who has successfully lost weight and kept the weight off, as well as raised their happiness quotient, exercised. No excuses. Period. But the benefits are so worth it that I promise you this habit is well worth adopting, no matter what your age, limitations or current physical fitness level.

Mary may have had hip problems, but that didn't keep her from swimming and doing strength training at the gym. She exchanged her excuses and dishonesty for a clear plan for getting her weight under control. By the end of the year, she'd lost 45 pounds:

"Most important and something I wasn't even expecting is that within weeks of cleaning up my eating act, I noticed that the grey cloud that had been hanging over my head for years began to lift. I started to feel like me again. I like that change even more than the weight loss. I'll never go back to my old eating habits. It's just not worth it!"

SECRET 1:
EAT REAL 75% OF THE TIME

The Promise

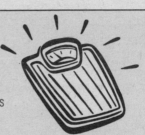

In one week of making this change, you will:

- lose a pound or two
- notice a drop in food cravings

In one month, you will:

- have more energy
- think more clearly
- notice improvements in memory and mood
- drop additional pounds
- notice more "joie de vivre" in your attitude

In one year, you will:

- lose up to 25 pounds (the more junk you eliminate and real foods you include, the more weight you will lose)
- feel and look 5 to 10 years younger
- lower your risk for all age-related diseases, including heart disease, cancer, diabetes, hypertension and memory loss

Sam's a new man since he learned an important lesson a few years back. That isn't his real name, but he was adamant that I not disclose his identity—he's a bit embarrassed about the story I'm about to tell. Just forget that I told you he is a marriage and family counselor living in Southern California and has McDreamy-like hair any woman worth her weight in estrogen would die to run her fingers through. Sam didn't always have that hair. In fact, it was almost losing those locks that taught him the lesson.

Sam ate reasonably well as long as Mom was cooking throughout his high school years, but the diet thing really took a nosedive when he flew the coop for college. With no one in the dorm cafeteria nagging him to eat vegetables, he slid through the first year of college living on pizza and Coke. His menu choices went from bad to worse once he moved into his own house. "There were days when all I ate was Costco muffins or Super Value meals," he admits, then adds, "Except my one-dish wonder—boxed mac 'n' cheese— I don't remember ever dirtying a pan."

For years, he appeared to get by eating these diet disasters, but somewhere around his late twenties the gig was up. "I was young, but I was losing my hair. I was having horrible stomach pains and I felt awful. Hey, I was starting to look like my dad, which isn't a bad thing except that he's 32 years older than me!" Around that time, a friend casually mentioned that no one could live on what Sam ate without dying a horrible death at a young age. It was a joke, but he took it to heart. It was just the wake-up call he needed. "I didn't cook, I hated vegetables and I was addicted to Cheez Whiz, but I also was scared," he recalls.

That is how I met Sam. He showed up at my office anxious but ready to make changes and without a clue where to start. He was sure I would force him to drink wheatgrass smoothies or dine on brewer's yeast muffins. Instead, we started small, just to get him used to eating real food. He began by snacking on oranges and bananas instead of chips and by buying roasted chickens and cartons of low-fat milk at the grocery store instead of pulling into a drive-through for his two millionth Big Mac. Next step was to eat more regularly and stock the kitchen with easy-to-make foods, like peanut butter, whole-grain breads, precut vegetables and frozen berries. "I found I didn't even need to cook to eat well," he says, "which was a huge relief for this kitchen-phobic guy."

The diet trend snowballed. The better he ate, the better he felt, and the better he felt, the more motivated he was to eat better. Within a few months, his hair was growing back and his stomach pains had vanished. It's been years since those diet-disaster days, and Sam is a born-again nutrition junkie.

Sam's story is not unique. From the science lab to my office, the results are always the same. A study from the University of California, Los Angeles, found that people showed significant improvements in memory and mental function within just two weeks of eating healthier. I can't tell you how many times people have told me similar stories. They followed my advice and were amazed at how much better they felt. Even people who think they eat well notice improvements in energy, mood, motivation, thinking ability, waistline measurements and more when they make additional changes in how, when and what they eat. I truly can't understand why people don't take better care of themselves, when the payoffs are so incredible!

But then, I'm also astounded by what people put up with. They tolerate feeling tired day in and day out. They shoulder depression or mood swings that strain relationships and dampen enjoyment of life. They give in to food cravings then blame themselves for being weak willed. They trudge through the day on little sleep and no enthusiasm. Their shoulders are tight from stress, their stomachs are in a knot and their brains are muddled. Often they look older than their years or are just plain worn-out. Maybe, like Sam, they are losing their hair, or their skin has lost its glow.

The food-mood issue can work to your advantage or against it. When you feel down, you eat worse, which only makes you feel lousier. That's what study after study has found, including one from the University of Southern California on air-traffic controllers, which found that stress snowballs into mood problems, like depression, which then leads to physical problems. The fatigue and depression leave you less motivated to eat well or take care of yourself. It might be all that you can do to drag yourself through the day. You may wind up lighting up, slugging down alcohol, vegging in front of the TV, eating junk and perhaps not even complying with instructions about medication. As a result, you gain weight, feel and sleep worse, stress out and enjoy life less.

Change your eating habits and I promise you will feel better, which starts the spiral working upward out of depression, toward a new you. The more improvements you make in what you eat, the faster and more dramatic the results.

We aren't meant to be in pain or depressed. We certainly are not designed to be fat. These are symptoms that something is wrong and needs fixing. Choosing real food and tossing the junk will help, if not solve, the problem.

What are Real Foods?

Real foods are authentic foods. They are foods as close to their original form as possible. They are the broccoli, not the broccoli in cheese sauce; the bowl of oatmeal, not the granola bar; and the berries, not the Flat Earth Wild Berry Patch Crisps. They are foods rich in all that Mother Nature designed them to be. They are naturally brimming with vitamins, minerals, fiber, essential fats, protein and the thousands and thousands of health-enhancing, antioxidant-rich phytochemicals that protect our brains and bodies from disease and aging. Real foods don't have ingredient lists, and when they do, you recognize and can pronounce everything on it. Real foods grow on trees, bushes or vines. They have two or four legs, or fins. You know them as plain fruits, vegetables, whole grains, legumes, lean meats or seafood, plain milk products, or foods made from these basic ingredients.

Where Do I Find Real Foods?

Check out the following sources to get you started on the search for real foods.

eatwellguide.org and **localharvest.org:** provide information on where to get grass-fed beef and organic produce.

organicconsumers.org: an eye-opener on how your shopping choices affect the environment.

wwoofusa.org: stands for Worldwide Opportunities on Organic Farms, USA; a chance to volunteer on an organic farm.

centerforfoodsafety.org: keeps you updated on government policies and provides a place to learn how you can influence Congress and other agencies to support a sustainable real-food supply.

The more humans tamper with real foods, the less nutritious they get, and the further they are from alive, fresh or nutrient-packed. In general, the more pro-cessed a food, the lower its vitamin, mineral, fiber and phytonutrient content and the higher its calories, fat, salt and sugar.

Processed grains, for example, are a nutritional wasteland. Most, if not all, of the original vitamins, minerals, antioxidants, phytonutrients and fiber have been stripped away when the germ and bran layers were removed from the whole wheat, leaving only the white, carb-filling inside. Then one measly mineral and four vitamins are added back to "enrich" these pathetic grains. And that's just the flour that goes into a processed food like the bun on a Big Mac, the flakes in most cereal boxes or the muffins, scones and pas-tries at Starbucks.

A friend of mine tried an experiment with a fast-food hamburger. She put it on a shelf, tucked away in her kitchen. Six months later, it looked almost exactly the same. That hamburger and bun were so processed, mold didn't even grow on it! A food that dead is not worth eating.

Five Real Foods to Limit

They might be natural, organic or real, but these foods are nutritional duds that will undermine your mood, health and waistline. Limit or avoid them.

- Butter
- Red meat with a fat content higher than 7% by weight
- Lard
- Egg yolks (no more than 6 a week)
- Full-fat cheese

Real Food, Not Sawdust

Real foods are the fuel on which humans evolved on. They are the diets that hunter-gatherers hunted and gathered for hundreds of thousands of years. Think about that the next time you bite into a cracker topped with cream cheese, stick your fork into a plateful of Hamburger Helper or quench your thirst with a bottle of Vitamin Water. None of these foods—or any processed food for that matter—ever passed the lips of even one of our ancient ancestors, dating back far before recorded history.

Real foods are like breathing in pure, clean, mountain-fresh, oxygen-rich air. Real foods are what our bodies need, not just to live, but to thrive. It is real food, alive with nutrients, that our bodies require to run like well-oiled machines. In contrast, diets filled with processed foods are as alien to our age-old bodies as breathing in carbon monoxide. It's no wonder that when people choose diets rich in real foods they rave about how great they feel—and we notice how great they look.

Here is the catch. It's not that real food is good for us. You wouldn't say that gasoline is good for a car or even that water is good for a fish. It's just that when our bodies don't get enough real food, they begin to break down, just as a car will sputter and stop when the tank is filled with dirty gasoline or a fish will die without a drink.

It was junk food that caused Sam's hair to fall out and it was real food that grew it back. It is processed food that leads to weight gain, depression and disease, and it is real food that lifts us out of the doldrums. When Sam turned to a diet based on real foods, his body was able to work in harmony with its natural rhythms and he started feeling great for the first time in years. He also looked great, lowered his disease risk, had more energy, lost weight effortlessly, started thinking more clearly and looked five years younger. Not bad for a minimal amount of effort in the kitchen department!

The Natural High

When we choose diets based on real foods, we work in tune with our natural rhythm and balance, which allows our bodies to grow, mend and thrive in ways far beyond our wildest dreams.

The Whole 9 Yards

I am frequently asked what foods will bless people with more energy or improve their moods, as if adding a mango or a bowl of flaxseed to an otherwise horrid diet is all it takes to turn the grump ship around. Granted, there are some mood-boosting superfoods that we will explore in Chapter 5, but they won't do you much good if your overall diet stinks. On the other hand, sprinkle those superfoods into a diet based on real foods and voilà! Miracles happen.

Thousands of studies spanning decades of research, including ones from the University of Toronto and Tufts University in Boston, repeatedly report that the more real foods people eat, the lower their disease risk and the happier and leaner they are. For example, cutting back on processed foods high in saturated fat lowers disease risk, but combine that habit with extra fruits and vegetables and disease risk drops significantly more. One study that followed

10,449 people for ten years found that those people who ate the most real food, such as fruits, vegetables and legumes, had the lowest risk of dying from any cause, including heart disease or cancer. The Centers for Disease Control and Prevention (CDC) report that people who skip the junk, avoid fast-food restaurants and instead focus on real food are the ones most successful at long-term weight loss.

The Mediterranean diet is a perfect example. This diet dramatically lowers disease risk and aids in long-term weight loss, and studies report that the closer people follow the Mediterranean diet, the happier they are. This traditional diet (which, by the way, is almost extinct and holds no resemblance to most meals you'll get today in Rome, Barcelona, Athens or Morocco) is based on grains (pasta, polenta and other whole grains), fruits, vegetables and legumes. It has a daily allotment for small amounts of olive oil and yogurt, while fish or poultry grace the plate a couple of times a week. Meat or sweets are eaten rarely, or a couple times a month. Wine, typically red wine, is consumed in moderation. Except for a few sweets and pasta, there are virtually no processed foods in this traditional diet.

What is the secret to the Mediterranean diet? You will get a different answer depending on which researcher you ask. Some experts vow it is the lycopene in the tomatoes that lowers disease risk. Others say it is the healthy fats in fish and olives along with all the antioxidants and anti-inflammatory phytonutrients in olive oil. The lack of saturated fat and the abundance of fiber-rich carbs also have been credited for the low risk of diabetes, depression, obesity, heart disease and cancer. The vitamin- and mineral-packed produce has been noted for improvements in mood, the high amount of lutein is thought to contribute to the low risk for vision loss, the resveratrol in the wine is certainly the reason why inflammatory diseases such as Alzheimer's are low, while the probiotics in the yogurt must explain why digestive tract problems are rare. Other researchers vow the high vitamin C and beta-carotene from all that produce explain why cancer rates are low, yet some studies conclude that the high magnesium intakes are the reason why stress levels are low. Recent studies from Arizona State University even suggest that the vinegar so prevalent in the salad dressings used in this region is the reason why obesity and arthritis are almost nonexistent.

In truth, you can't isolate one factor out of tens of thousands. It is the perfect amount and balance of the 40+ nutrients mixed with close to a million phytonutrients that are supplied only by a diet based on real food. It is that balance on which our bodies depend. It is that balance that allows our immune, antioxidant and cell communication systems to keep the ship, our bodies, running in tip-top condition. It is the entire diet, not one food or one nutrient. In fact, the Mediterranean diet is just one of several real-foods diets, from the Okinawan diet based on an eating style associated with extreme longevity to vegetarian or Asian cuisines, all of which are loaded with real foods and skimpy on processed junk. That is the secret to long, healthy, happy lives and fit bodies. It's the whole package, and the whole package needs to be mostly real, not processed.

Of course, happy, fit people know this. They might not have begun their journey intending to cut out processed foods. Many found along the way, as they experimented, failed and succeeded, that they were most successful at weight loss and were happiest in the process when they minimized the tempting junk.

Alex, a college student in Washington, experienced this firsthand:

"In high school, I went all out on greasy, sugary, processed stuff. I ate pizza for lunch, rewarded myself with ice cream every night, nibbled on sugary snacks and salty foods like chips, drank soft drinks and ordered the croissant along with the Starbucks whole-milk peppermint mocha with whip. It's no surprise why I continuously gained weight in high school! Two years ago, I decided I needed a major diet overhaul. I put a lid on the processed stuff. I switched to salads, chicken breast, whole grains, nonfat

MEDITERRANEAN DIET PYRAMID

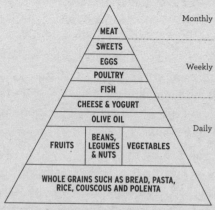

MEAT — Monthly

SWEETS
EGGS
POULTRY — Weekly
FISH

CHEESE & YOGURT
OLIVE OIL — Daily

FRUITS | BEANS, LEGUMES & NUTS | VEGETABLES

WHOLE GRAINS SUCH AS BREAD, PASTA, RICE, COUSCOUS AND POLENTA

Daily Beverage Recommendations:
6 Glasses of Water • Wine in moderation

OKINAWA DIET PYRAMID

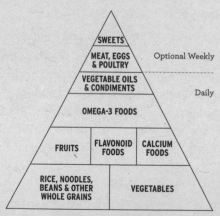

SWEETS

MEAT, EGGS & POULTRY — Optional Weekly

VEGETABLE OILS & CONDIMENTS — Daily

OMEGA-3 FOODS

FRUITS | FLAVONOID FOODS | CALCIUM FOODS

RICE, NOODLES, BEANS & OTHER WHOLE GRAINS | VEGETABLES

Daily Beverage Recommendations:
Tea • Alcohol in moderation

VEGETARIAN DIET PYRAMID

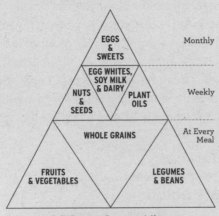

Daily Beverage Recommendations:
6 Glasses of Water • Alcohol in moderation

ASIAN DIET PYRAMID

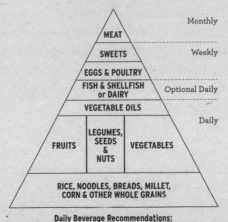

Daily Beverage Recommendations:
6 Glasses of Water or Tea • Sake, Wine, Beer in moderation

sugar-free lattes instead of the peppermint mochas, tons of vegetables and drank lots of water. What a difference it made in my energy level and my weight! I lost 60 pounds, and I've kept it off. And my energy level is so much higher. I'm more confident and I love my life. I cannot even imagine what my life would be like right now if I hadn't made a conscious decision to change."

Need I say more?

The 75% Solution

By now I hope I've convinced you to reexamine your diet and see where you can switch from processed to real foods. You don't have to give up everything. Like Sam, who still eats pizza and pastries, you can include foods that come in a box, bag or wrapper. Just aim for a diet where real food outweighs the processed stuff. If three out of every four foods you choose is a real food, or if three out of every four bites comes from a food straight off the vine, bush or plant, then you should be eating authentically enough to guarantee a better mood and a thinner waistline.

It's the 75% solution—75% of everything that goes into your mouth should be a real food. This solution allows you to live in this toxic environment of fast-food restaurants and more than 45,000 processed items on the grocery shelves, yet be happier and thinner.

The 75% solution makes it easy to eat right without spending hours in the kitchen or sacrificing taste and enjoyment. Check out "The Real-Foods Shopping List" on page 15 for the types of foods to focus on when shopping. Even when purchasing processed foods, look for ones with the most real ingredients. For example, follow the rules outlined in Chapter 3 when searching for processed foods with the most whole grains. For other foods, here are a few guidelines:

1. Total fat: 3 grams fat/100 calories. That is the limit for fat in processed foods. Shelve any product that has more fat than that. You want foods that are low in fat (especially saturated and trans fats), supply some fiber and pack a low to moderate calorie punch. The more fat, the more calories. So limit total fat to no more than 3 grams/100 calories.

The focus is on fat ratios, rather than fat grams, because you don't want to reward companies that keep the fat grams low by serving up tiny portions. A label on a frozen entree might say, "Only 8 grams of fat and 210 calories," but is that really a meal? One cup of fruited yogurt has 250 calories and we don't call that a meal. It's a snack. True, almost 7 out of every 10 Americans are battling a weight problem, but even diets shouldn't drop below 1,200 calories a day; if people eat a third of their calories at each meal, that means at least 400 calories. Eat a 200-calorie entree and you're likely to say, "Hey, that meal was so healthy, I can have a little treat now, like that half gallon of ice cream in the freezer." What you want is a meal that will fill you up with healthy food without filling you out with too many calories.

2. *Limit saturated fat to 1 gram saturated fat/100 calories.* Look for items that have less than 10% of calories from saturated fat. That means about 1 gram of saturated fat or less for every 100 calories.

3. *No trans fats.* Sure, the label says in big, bold print: "NO TRANS FATS." But "zero" trans fats aren't always zero. It might mean 0.5 milligrams in labelese. Check the ingredient list for "hydrogenated vegetable oils." If you see it, shelve it. An exception to this rule is peanut butter. There is so little hydrogenated fat in most peanut butters that it would take 153 servings (for a total of 28,764 calories!) to get even 0.5 milligrams of trans fats.

4. *Limit sodium.* Whether you have high blood pressure or not, you can benefit by cutting back on your sodium intake. Many processed foods, particularly the frozen breakfast and dinner entrees, packaged grains, meals in a can or bag and, of course, snack foods, are sodium land mines, supplying up to a full day's maximum allotment for sodium, which is 2,400 milligrams. Look for real foods that are close to sodium free, then complement these foods with packaged items that have no more than 480 milligrams per serving.

Happy, Fit People's Tricks of the Trade

The cross-country runners I counseled at both Ohio State and the University of Oregon lost weight on 7,000 calories a day. Don't you wish you could indulge in anything you wanted to eat just like a 20-year-old who runs 100 miles a week?! Well, forget it. For the rest of us—skinny or fat, young or old, male or female—we must put a lid on our calorie intake or expect to end up sad and fat. Here are some tricks happy, fit people have shared with me over the years that help them stay lean and upbeat:

"Order salads without the croutons or cheese, and with the dressing on the side. Leave 95% of the dressing behind when the salad is done."

"At restaurants, ask that your toast be served dry, no butter. Also, ask the waiter to cancel the baked potato or fries and give you a double order of steamed veggies."

"Use mustard, not mayonnaise, on sandwiches."

"I save hundreds of dollars and scads of calories by bringing my own water bottle, rather than purchasing colas, bottled teas or sports drinks."

"Never eat anything that is breaded or fried."

"My most important diet rule is that I can't eat unless the meal includes at least two fruits and vegetables."

"Brush your teeth after dinner and you'll be less tempted to snack in the evening."

"When I eat out, I ask the waiter to doggie-bag half my entree before it comes to the table."

"I eat breakfast at dinnertime, which leaves me less tempted to want dessert."

"Either lunch or dinner every day is a salad."

"I pack my own lunch and snacks. That way I know what and how much I'm eating."

"When I'm tempted to eat some junk food, I remind myself that it will take 5 minutes to eat it, then I'll be right back where I started, only feeling guilty and maybe stuffed."

"I chew gum whenever I'm tempted to overeat, like when I'm cooking so I don't taste test or after a meal when I can hear the cookies calling to me."

A Real-Foods Diet à la Packaged Foods

Here are a few examples of how you can mix real foods with processed foods for the 75% solution to balance optimal nutrition with the reality of a fast-paced life.

BREAKFAST

Option 1: A whole-grain waffle. Look for one that supplies at least 3 grams of fiber. Top it with peanut butter and thawed frozen blueberries. Serve with calcium- and vitamin D–fortified orange juice.

Option 2: Lean Pockets Bacon, Egg & Cheese. This meets the criteria for fat and saturated fat but is a bit high in sodium, so serve it with a bowl of fruit canned in its own juice and a glass of calcium-fortified grapefruit juice. (Read labels on fruit juice: a label can say 100% fruit juice, but if that juice comes from pear, white grape or apple concentrates, all you have is sugar water. Look for juices that do not contain these concentrates and don't contain high fructose corn syrup. Your best bets are 100% orange juice, pineapple juice and tomato juice. See Chapter 8 for more on beverages.)

Option 3: A veggie omelet. Make it with leftover vegetables and egg substitute mixed with one whole egg. Serve with toasted whole wheat bread, a glass of 1% milk and half a cantaloupe.

Option 4: A bowl of oatmeal. Try the Plum Nuts Oatmeal or Pumpkin Pie Oatmeal from the Recipes section or Quaker Simple Harvest Instant Multigrain Hot Cereal cooked in milk or soy milk. Serve with a glass of 100% calcium- and vitamin D–fortified orange juice.

LUNCH

Option 1: A Kashi Veggie Medley. Serve with a clamshell of cut-up fruit from the produce department and a glass of soy milk or tub of Rachel's Yogurt with DHA.

Option 2: Shrimp cocktail. Try a container of thawed cooked shrimp with cocktail sauce from the freezer case. Serve with baby carrots and low-fat dip, apple slices, tossed salad or other fruits/vegetables. Or just buy cooked frozen shrimp and toss with bagged lettuce for an instant lunch salad.

Option 3: Frozen pizzas. This one is a bit tricky, but you can have your pizza and maintain your waistline and mood, too. In general, go for the pizzas with the most vegetables. For example, a slice of Essensia Pizza Spinach Mushroom Classic Vegetable or of Freschetta Roasted Portabella Mushrooms and Spinach has up to 100 calories less per slice and much less fat and saturated fat of any pizza made with only cheese or cheese and meat. Or try the Kashi whole-grain pizzas. They don't quite fit the fat, saturated fat and/or sodium limits, but they are close and the crust is whole grain. Serve with a big tossed salad with low-fat bottled dressing. Also, doctor your pizza by adding sliced tomatoes or frozen pepper slices. Watch out for the serving sizes when you're reading and comparing pizza labels.

Option 4: Canned soups. Foods with the word "healthy" in their title, such as Campbell's Healthy Request soups, must abide by standards for fat, saturated fat and sodium, so it's a sure sign the food is really and truly healthier. Doctor your soup and dilute the sodium even more by adding extra frozen or leftover vegetables. For example, up until third grade, my kids did not know that Campbell's Chicken Noodle Soup didn't come without peas. Serve any soup with fresh fruit and a bagged salad.

DINNER

How does a person sift out the bad from the good?

Let's focus on one department, the freezer case. Frozen-food entrees have come a long way since the days of TV dinners and the choice between meatloaf or fried chicken. First they trimmed the fat, thanks to lines like Lean Cuisine. Then Healthy Choices led the troops in cutting the salt. Now Lean Cuisine's Spa Cuisine, Kashi, Barbara's and Amy's, to name a few, have added whole grains. Some add a smattering of vegetables, though none add enough. In most cases, you can measure the vegetables in teaspoons, not cups. The good news is you can get lots of veggies in the frozen-food aisle to complement your frozen dinner.

Option 1: Beef. Salisbury Steak remains an all-time favorite, which can make or break your health depending on the choice. Remember the 3 grams of fat and about 1 gram of saturated fat for every 100 calories rules. With these guidelines in mind, Healthy Choices and, believe it or not, Hungry Man both meet the criteria, although both are very high in sugar, supplying about 5 teaspoons of sugar for a dinner! In contrast, others, such as Claim Jumper's version, can pack in more than 600 calories, with 50% of it coming from fat and more than 3 teaspoons of saturated fat. Serve the Healthy Choice or Hungry Man with steamed frozen vegetables, such as green peas or green beans, and a tossed salad made from bagged lettuce and low-fat dressing. Banquet Crock-Pot Classics Stroganoff Beef & Noodles or Beef Stew, Lean Cuisine Café Classics Teriyaki Steak and Lean Cuisine Dinnertime Selections Steak Tips also Dijon all meet the criteria for fat and saturated fat.

Option 2: Pasta. A quick-fix dinner could include whole-grain pasta topped with spaghetti sauce and served with steamed, frozen vegetables and a bagged tossed salad. Unfortunately, this is one place where carbs have gotten their bad name. Not because pasta has a lot of calories, but because so many pasta entrees are laden with fat. You could have more than five Garlic Beef and Broccoli frozen entrees for the calories in one Marie Callender's Fettucine Alfredo with Garlic Bread. On the other hand, Kashi Chicken Pasta Pomodor is a great choice. Again, serve with steamed frozen vegetables and a salad to round out the meal.

Option 3: Chicken. There are lots of choices here, including any Healthy Choices, Weight Watchers, or Lean Cuisine Café or Spa Cuisine Classic chicken entree. Serve with bagged salad, frozen vegetables, and a glass of 1% milk.

Option 4: Seafood. Fish is good for you. It's the only natural dietary source of the omega-3 fat, DHA (docosahexaenoic acid), which lowers your risk for heart disease and possibly bone loss, depression, memory loss and more. Lean Cuisine Spa Cuisine Classic Salmon with Basil is a great choice and one of the few entrees on the market to supply those healthy omega-3s!

You even can have dessert on a real-food diet. Dole Fruit Juice Bars have only 30 calories and little sugar. Mrs. Smith's Hearty Pumpkin Pie and Pumpkin Custard Pie and Mrs. Smith's Reduced Fat, No Sugar Added Apple Pie are the healthiest pie selections in the frozen food case. The very best frozen dessert of all is fresh or frozen fruit (check out Chapter 4 for tons of ideas). For me, it is frozen blueberries. They taste like sorbet, but have no added sugar and pack a huge antioxidant punch!

Put Real Back into Your Cupboards

I'm well aware that for some people switching to a real-foods diet will take some effort. But that doesn't mean you can't do it. We all do things we don't want to do or that are hard. Hey, who wants to pay taxes or get up in the morning?!

Happy, fit people work at it, too. Any person over the age of 25 who is happy and fit is working on it, trust me. They plan, organize, prepare and set limits and rules. They monitor what, when and how much they eat. Granted, it takes more time and discipline to plan meals around real food than it does to take medication for diabetes or heart disease, but the pay-offs are so amazing! For a little delayed gratification of saying "no" to a doughnut today, you lose weight, feel great, have more energy, think more clearly, look younger and feel vibrant tomorrow.

Here are the three most powerful habits you can adopt to make the transition from a diet that fuels the flames of depression and weight gain to one that helps you get back on track weight- and mood-wise.

Habit #1: Purge your kitchen. The more junk-food temptation you can remove from your house, the better off you will be. Clear out the junk so it won't control your life.

Habit #2: Restock the fort. Once the cupboards are bare, restock with real foods, using the "The Real-Foods Shopping List" below and the "100+ Products That Meet Most of the Real-Food Guidelines" on page 425 as a guide. You need to feel full and satisfied to be happy and willing to stick with any weight-loss eating plan. Studies show that anything short of this leads to anxiety, stress and depression. So make sure you always have tasty but good-for-you foods around.

Habit #3: Bring foods with you. Never leave the house without packing a lunchbag, your briefcase, purse, glove compartment or diaper or gym bag with real foods, such as apple slices, peanuts, a thermos of soup or smoothie, Triscuits and string cheese, a sandwich on 100% whole-grain bread, and so on.

The Real-Foods Shopping List

PRODUCE: FRUITS & VEGETABLES

In the Produce Department: All fresh fruits and vegetables; fresh herbs

Down the Aisles: Fruits canned in their own juices; bottled 100% orange, grapefruit, tomato or prune juice; dried fruit; canned tomatoes: paste, stewed or whole; low-fat marinara sauce; salsa

In the Refrigerator Case: Cartons of 100% orange or grapefruit juice

In the Freezer Case: Plain vegetables (not potatoes); fruit such as berries, peaches and cherries

GRAINS/CEREALS

In the Bakery: 100% whole grains: breads, bagels, English muffins, pita bread, rolls and tortillas

Down the Aisles: Wheat germ, corn or whole-wheat tortillas; whole-wheat crackers, such as Triscuits; air-popped popcorn; rice: brown (instant or regular), Brown basmati or texmati, Wehani or wild rice; hot cereals, such as rolled oats, Kashi, bulgar, quinoa, barley, and Quaker Simple Harvest Instant Multi-grain Hot Cereal; whole-grain ready-to-eat cereals, such as Shredded Wheat, NutriGrain, Post Whole-Wheat Raisin Bran, GrapeNuts, low-fat granola, Puffed Kashi; pasta, such as whole-wheat or whole-wheat-blend noodles; flour, such as whole-wheat, rye, oat

In the Freezer Case: Whole-grain waffles

MEAT, FISH, AND LEGUMES

In the Meat Department: Extra-lean cuts (no more than 7% fat by weight); poultry breast; all seafood (except tilapia, which is low in omega-3 and high in omega-6 fats)

Down the Aisles: Canned tuna, clams, or salmon, packed in water (limit intake of tuna to no more than 6 ounces/week because of mercury); all dried beans and peas, including kidney, black, garbanzo, navy, soybean, lentils, split peas and lima; canned cooked dried beans and peas (beans in prepared "dishes" such as chili or baked beans should be chosen on an individual basis by their fat and sodium content); packaged bean mixes, such as hummus and lentil pilaf (check sodium content); nut butters, including peanut, almond, soy and cashew, preferably "natural" versions; fat-free refried beans

In the Produce Department: Tofu: silken, firm and extra-firm

MILK & OTHER HIGH-CALCIUM ITEMS

In the Dairy Case: 1% or nonfat milk; plain low-fat or nonfat yogurt; nonfat buttermilk, DHA-fortified soy milk; fat-free or low-fat cottage cheese; low-fat cheeses; fresh mozzarella cheese; soy cheese; fat-free or low-fat ricotta cheese; fat-free cream cheese; fat-free sour cream; fat-free half & half; fat-free whipped cream; eggs or egg substitutes; calcium- and vitamin D–fortified orange or grapefruit juice.

OILS & FATS

Down the Aisles: Olive oil; nut oils; fat-free or low-calorie salad dressing; salad spritzers; fat-free or low-calorie mayonnaise

SWEETS & DESSERTS

Down the Aisles: Jam; honey; baby food prunes (as fat replacement in recipes); cookies made from 100% whole grains

In the Freezer Case: Frozen 100% fruit bars and fruit ices; low-fat ice creams & sorbets

CONDIMENTS

Down the Aisles: Vinegars; mustards; baker's yeast; herbs and spices

How Much?

Lisa is 5'3" tall and at least 60 pounds overweight. She swears she only eats grilled chicken breasts, vegetables and whole grains. Rollie and Dolores enjoy gourmet meals, with lots of real foods, but they also go through more calorie-packed olive oil in a month than I use in a year. Both are as fit as fiddles, lean, happy and in great health.

What's going on here? Granted, Lisa has a slight honesty issue to address, since no one can be that overweight without eating something a bit more calorific. However, it also shows that it's not just what we eat, but how much. Lisa eats in quantity, far more than she needs, while Rollie and Dolores revel in small amounts of highly flavorful delicacies. Eat too much of almost anything—even healthy, real foods—and you gain weight.

Portions have ballooned ten-fold in the past 30 years, both inside and outside the home, with the greatest increases in processed fast food, foods high in refined carbs and meat. Restaurants are using larger plates, bakers are selling bigger muffin tins, pizzerias are using larger pans, cars have larger cup holders and fast-food restaurants are packaging drinks and French fries in bigger containers. A study from the University of North Carolina found these bigger portions mean extra calories, while U.S. Department of Agriculture (USDA) reports the average American has added up to 300 extra calories a day compared to intakes back in the mid-1980s.

Big meals and huge portions also leave you feeling sluggish, which is a big no-no if you want to be happy and energetic. "I have so much more energy, more motivation to get all the tasks done on my daily to-do list, and just feel more alive if I don't overeat," says Vince, a personal trainer in Oregon. He found that if he pushes back from the table when he is still slightly hungry, it makes all the difference in his energy level. "It takes a bit of willpower to stop shoveling food into my mouth when I'm not yet stuffed, and sometimes I have to keep myself busy for the next 15 to 20 minutes after a meal to avoid diving into the cookie jar, but then I feel so much better the rest of the day and evening that it is absolutely worth it!"

We all must get real about portions. People always, and I mean always, underestimate how much they eat, especially when it comes to grains, meat and fast food. The heavier we are, the more we fudge the numbers. In fact, we typically fail to admit to about 700 calories a day! John Foreyt, Ph.D., Director of the Behavioral Medicine Research Center at Baylor College of Medicine in Houston, Texas, and an expert on weight management, says the dishonesty issue is so prevalent that he factors it into his diet consults. "People typically underestimate their overall food intake by about a third, so for people to be truly honest about their calorie balance, I recommend they keep food journals then add at least a third more calories to their daily total."

Happy, fit people have learned that being your own portion police pays off. Maureen, a freelance writer in Portland, Oregon, lost 30 pounds by cutting back on portions and focusing on real foods:

> "I found I was just as satisfied with smaller portions every two to three hours instead of bigger meals. If I loaded up on lots of fiber, I felt full, so I was less apt to overeat. Then I took the big step and started experimenting with healthy recipes that were super easy to make (I am not a good cook, don't like to cook, and will not spend a lot of time on it). I also started bringing healthy, quick snacks with me, like veggies with white bean hummus. Just those little efforts paid off big-time!"

Portion Precision

To get real about portions, buy a scale and a measuring cup and take one week practicing how to accurately identify a portion. For example,

Extra-lean meat, chicken, fish	3 ounces or the size of a deck of cards or the palm of a woman's hand
Whole grain pasta, rice, oatmeal, potatoes, cooked vegetables	½ cup or the size of your fist or a tennis ball

Whole grain bagel or muffin	1 ounce or the size of a ping pong ball
Low-fat cheese	1 ounce or the size of a woman's thumb
Olive oil	1 teaspoon or the size of a stamp
Low-calorie salad dressing	2 tablespoons or the size of a standard ice cube
Raw vegetables or fruit	cup or the size of a baseball

Dining Out Needn't Do You In

Never before in the history of the planet have so many people dined out as often as they do today. In an effort to edge out the competition, restaurants offer megasized servings. These "value meals" are extra-heavy on the fat and calories. It's no wonder that body weight and depression rates increase in direct proportion to how often a person dines out, especially when those meals are from fast-food chains.

According to the USDA, a serving of meat should be 3 ounces. But at your typical restaurant, whether it's a steak or the turkey on your deli sandwich, the meat can weigh up to 16 ounces. That's more than five servings! Reduce that portion from 16 ounces to 3 ounces and save yourself up to 1,200 calories.

Refined grains are another food we have come to expect in megaportions. According to the USDA and its Pyramid Food Guide, we should include 5 to 11 servings of grain in our daily diets. A serving of pasta is ½ cup, which is about four fork twirls. (Granted, most people eat more than this, so perhaps one cup or two servings of pasta would be a realistic portion.) Most pasta dishes in restaurants are served as platters, not portions, and average four or more cups. Add the garlic bread and you have two to three days' worth of grains in one meal.

The solution? Regardless of what's on the plate, it's up to you to take charge of how much you eat. Request half orders, order à la carte or bag half your entree before you begin to eat. A recent study found that eating your salad first (and without the dressing) fills you up so you cut your portion of the main course and save yourself calories. Besides, that salad is a perfect place to tally up some super mood foods. (See Chapter 5 for which ones those are.)

Many of us are in a hurry and grab food on the go. How does this influence portions? Just assume that the portion of anything you eat at a fast-food establishment is too big and packs two to five times more calories than you ever would imagine. Coffee only comes in tall, grande and humongous (what ever happened to small and regular?); the Starbucks Grande White Chocolate mocha contains 470 calories and almost 5 teaspoons of fat, which is the calorie equivalent of eating a huge piece of chocolate devil's food cake with frosting.

Fast-casual restaurants are all the rage now. Baja Fresh is an example of a Mexican food chain that has a wonderful salsa bar. But their Dos Manos Enchilada-Style Burrito weighs 62 ounces and contains 3,370 calories, 39 teaspoons of fat, and 63 grams of saturated fat! Even if you only ate once a day, you'd gain weight on that meal!

The solution? You can have your mocha and drink it, too. Just order a tall made with nonfat milk, skip the whipped cream, top it with a few chocolate shavings and sweeten with aspartame or Splenda. When it comes to the burrito at Baja Fresh, order the Vegetarian Bare Burrito (for 560 calories) and split it with a partner.

Also, don't be fooled by the so-called healthier options at fast-food chains. They can present even bigger portion and calorie problems than the typical fare. For example,

- A Smoked Turkey Club Sandwich at Au Bon Pain contains 760 calories and 34 grams of fat (8.5 teaspoons!).
- Burger King's BK Big Fish Sandwich supplies 710 calories and 39 grams of fat, half of which are saturated.
- A Crispy Chicken Caesar Salad at McDonald's with croutons and a packet of dressing supplies 550 calories, the calorie equivalent of a Quarter Pounder with Cheese and half of your day's allotment of fat (35.5 grams or 9 teaspoons).

The solution? At the drive-through, order grilled chicken breast sandwiches with no mayo and a glass of OJ, or split a burger and bring baby carrots and soy milk from home to accompany the meal. When it comes to fast-food salads, stick with grilled chicken, skip the croutons and ask for fat-free dressing.

When dining out, follow these rules:

1. The Unit Rule. The bigger the container, the more we eat. According to research at the University of Pennsylvania, people eat in units, such as a sandwich, a cookie, a plate of food, a bag of chips, a slice of pizza. Today, these units are jumbo burgers, bigger plates and muffins the size of small cakes. One way to overcome this problem is to request a half portion and have it served on a salad plate, instead of a dinner plate. Also, skip the "value" meals and "economy-sized" bags of munchies, share a small bag of candy at the theater instead of having a large bag all to yourself, get used to leaving food on your plate and order a kid's hamburger instead of the Big Mac.

2. Split an Entree. Share an entree and order side salads and soups to round out the meal.

3. Attitude Adjustment. In the past, eating out was a special occasion, so we gave ourselves license to eat what we wanted. Today, we average more than four meals a week away from home. That devil-may-care attitude doesn't work when the treats come so fast and furious. Either start considering restaurant fare as part of your healthy way of eating, or save your precious dollars and reserve restaurant meals for a once-a-month special occasion, not a weekly routine.

4. Load Up on Veggies. You don't have to eat less to downsize portions, just eat better. It's not bigger portions that cause weight problems, it's bigger portions of foods high in fat, sugar and calories. Help yourself to buckets of super mood foods, like vegetables, broth-based soups, fruits, whole grains, soy milk and other real foods high in water and fiber, and you will fill up before you fill out.

When to Eat Real Foods

It is not just *what* or even *how much,* but also *when* you eat that affects mood. Dieting, skipping meals or eating too few carbohydrates can lower blood sugar, with symptoms such as weakness, irritability and fatigue. Erratic eating habits cause blood sugar to drop, so the body runs out of energy just like a cell phone you forget to recharge. A study from the University of Bristol found that in a group of 144 adults, those who ate regularly, starting with breakfast, had the best moods, worked more efficiently and felt calmer at the end of the testing period compared to people who ate erratically or skipped meals.

People who divide their food intake into little meals and snacks throughout the day think more clearly and feel better than people who eat irregularly. In contrast, meal skippers are more prone to mood swings, probably because once they do eat, they eat too much of all the wrong stuff. People often think they can save calories by skipping meals, but if they kept food journals they'd find that they more than make up for those saved calories at other times of the day.

Recharge on a regular basis by eating nutritious little meals or snacks spaced every four or five hours throughout the day, starting with breakfast. Keep meals light. Heavy meals laden with fat or calories make you groggy during the day and undermine a good night's sleep, so you wake up cranky. In contrast, light meals of carbohydrate-rich fruits, vegetables, whole grains and legumes, with small amounts of protein-rich nonfat milk products and extra-lean meat are energizing.

Lunchables

I'll fill you in on breakfast in Chapter 2. Right now, let's do lunch.

As part of the "eat regularly" rule, stop midday to refuel. Make sure lunch contains some fat. A neurotransmitter called galanin rises at about the lunch hour and is at the helm of our appetite center, tickling our fancies for fat. The more fat we eat, the more galanin we produce. Order a cheeseburger and French fries or a tossed salad smothered in high-fat dressing, and your galanin levels are jammed into high gear, possibly leading to cravings for more fatty foods later in the day. You definitely need some fat to keep galanin happy, especially the good fats, like the healthy fats in nuts and olive oil and the omega-3 fat DHA in fish. So get some, but not too much, at the midday meal.

Don't make the mistake of focusing solely on carbs. A high-carbohydrate lunch, such as a plate of pasta with marinara sauce and a tossed salad, raises brain levels of the nerve chemical serotonin, which leaves you relaxed and perhaps a bit sleepy. This is fine if it is Saturday and you have nothing to do, but it could be disastrous if you are on a work deadline midweek.

10 Days' Worth of Mood-Boosting, Waist-Shrinking Lunch Ideas

1. **Wrap It:** Fill a Mission Life Balance flour tortilla with 2 ounces of turkey breast meat, ½ cup shredded romaine lettuce, 2 tablespoons grated carrot and 1 tablespoon low-fat Caesar salad dressing. Serve with a glass of 1% milk and a piece of fruit.

2. **Salad Fixings:** Top 3 cups of baby spinach and/or romaine lettuce with ½ cup berries, 1 tablespoon pecans, ½ cup broccoli florets, ⅓ cup kidney or black beans and 2 tablespoons low-fat dressing. Serve with 100% whole-grain bread and a slice of low-fat cheese.

3. **Pocket It:** Fill a 100% whole-wheat pita with ½ cup black beans, ¼ cup grated carrot, ¼ cup chopped cucumber, ¼ cup diced red peppers and 2 tablespoons light Italian salad dressing. Serve with Rachel's yogurt and a glass of 100% juice.

4. **Burgerville:** Top a 100% whole-wheat burger bun with a vegetarian burger, 2 tablespoons low-fat crumbled feta cheese, ⅓ cup baby spinach leaves, and 1 teaspoon Dijon mustard. Serve with a piece of fruit and a glass of 1% milk.

5. **Chicken of the Sea Sandwich:** Top 2 slices of 100% whole-grain bread with 2 large romaine lettuce leaves and a mixture of

2 ounces drained, water-packed tuna, 1 tablespoon balsamic vinegar, 1 tablespoon fat-free mayo and ¼ cup diced celery. Serve with a side salad or piece of fruit and a glass of soy milk.

6. Take-out Desperado: If you must go, then order a kid's cheeseburger, a side salad with fat-free dressing and apple dippers, or Wendy's Ultimate Chicken Grill Sandwich (hold the mayo), a carton of low-fat milk and a Mandarin Orange cup.

7. Soup 'n' Sandwich: Have a bowl of Campbell's Healthy Request Savory Chicken and Long Grain Rice soup and add extra frozen vegetables. Serve with fresh fruit and a grilled cheese sandwich made with 2 slices of 100% whole-grain bread, low-fat cheese and cooking spray instead of butter or oil.

8. Veggie Broil: Cut in half and toast a 100% whole-grain English muffin. On one side, put 2 tablespoons mashed avocado, ¼ cup alfalfa sprouts, 1 thin slice red onion, 1 teaspoon sesame seeds and 2 teaspoons low-fat ranch dressing, and top with 1 ounce grated, low-fat cheddar cheese. Place under broiler and heat until cheese bubbles. Remove and add other side of muffin to form a sandwich. Serve with tomato juice and a side salad or fruit.

9. Campfire Crunch Sandwich: Mix 2 tablespoons fat-free cream cheese with a dash of lemon juice, lemon peel, 2 tablespoons dried tart cherries, ¼ cup grated carrot and 3 tablespoons trail mix. Pile onto a slice of 100% whole-grain bread, spread evenly and top with second piece of bread to form a sandwich. Serve with 1% milk and a piece of fruit or a salad.

10. Bagel Sandwich and Slaw: Spread 2 teaspoons Dijon mustard on half a 100% whole-wheat bagel; layer red onion, cucumber, red pepper slices, spinach leaves and low-fat cheese; and top with the other half of the bagel. Serve with broccoli slaw made with broccoli-coleslaw mix, low-fat coleslaw dressing and dried cranberries.

The What, How Much, and When of Real Food

Real food is the foundation of a diet for a *natural high*. Happy, fit people get real. And the more real they get, the better they feel. Eat at least 75% of your foods as real foods; eat forkfuls, not forklift-fuls; and eat regularly throughout the day and I promise you will feel better and drop weight. In turn, that will improve your mood and motivate you to stick with the program, which means more weight loss and an even better, more even mood.

SECRET 2:
FOLLOW THE 1-2-3 RULE

The Promise

In one week of making this change, you will:

- notice improvements in energy level

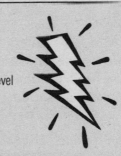

In one month, you will:

- think more clearly
- remember more
- have more consistent energy throughout the day
- notice a lessening of midday food cravings

In one year, you will:

- lose 15 pounds or more

I should have known better. I must have needed a kick in the head, because on a sunny day in the Napa Valley in California, I learned the hard way what happens when you don't eat the right breakfast.

My friend Karen and I were on our annual one-week bike trip. For the previous three days, we'd logged about 150 miles pedaling from the town of Sonoma to the oceanfront town of Bodega Bay (remember that Hitchcock movie *The Birds?*), up and down the coast, inland along the Russian River, and into a sweet little town called Healdsburg. (I'm telling you the route so you'll get an idea just how pooped our muscles were by the fourth day.) The owner of the B and B where we stayed prided herself as somewhat of a gourmet cook, so instead of the all-carb breakfast we needed (picture a big bowl of Shredded Wheat, nonfat milk, whole-wheat toast with jam, and fruit, then a second helping of cereal, maybe even a third), Chef B and B served us eggs Benedict, sausage, fried potatoes and fruit drowning in a goopy cream sauce. We scraped off the eggs and sauce, pushed the greasy potatoes and sausage aside, drained the cream, then ate what was left—the half English muffin and the fruit. Grumbling something about how anyone could eat that much grease and cholesterol, these two dietitians headed out for an all-day bike-a-thon. Ten miles short of our destination, we both hit "the wall."

You've heard about the wall, right? That's where athletes run or bicycle or swim long enough that they deplete their body's entire supply of quick-burning fuel, called glycogen. Once the fuel is gone, their muscles stop working.

Karen and I are anything but athletes, but we were definitely biting dust big-time at the wall. Now our muscles refused to move, our moods plummeted, and we were stuck on the highway without an ounce of motivation to move an inch, let alone 10 miles. Oh, and did I mention it was getting dark? "I'm not going any farther," Karen screamed at me, teeth bared and feet planted firmly off the bike and in the ditch. "We can't camp here," I whimpered. "Well, you can't make me move another inch either," she sputtered, nearly hitting me with her knapsack.

Needless to say, we did finish, but those were the longest and worst 10 miles of our lives. It was only after big platters of pasta that Karen and I could start being civil to each other again or even hobble to the hotel room. The conversation over dinner? The high-carb breakfast we had failed to eat that morning.

Granted, that is an extreme example and you might say, "Nice story, but I would drive, not bike, through the wine country. So what's the point?" The point is, we all need to refuel every morning to lesser or greater degrees. The consequences of not doing so leaves an athlete in the dust, but it also leaves the rest of us facing our own mini walls, from a lousy mood and muddled mind to a midday craving for chips and a thickening waistline down the road. Happy, fit people know better. Almost every single one of them makes sure to eat breakfast most, if not all, days of the week.

Why Breakfast Is a Natural High

Eating breakfast works with your body's natural rhythm, starting with your brain. That little computer sitting on top of your shoulders accounts for only 2% of your total body weight but gobbles as much as 30% of the calories you consume. It also is fuel fussy, demanding only glucose, which you get from starches and grains.

Of course, the rest of the body cries for carbs, too. By morning, it has been 8 to 12 hours since you last ate. During that time, the immediate fuel stores, called *glycogen* in your liver and muscle and *glucose* in your blood, have been used to keep the ol' body and brain machine ticking. Every second since that last meal, your body has been dipping into glucose stores to power your eyes blinking, hair growing, enzymes humming, brain dreaming, heart pumping and the other 43 kajillion processes, right down to making sure that taco you had for dinner has been digested, absorbed and used to build tissues.

I bet you seldom go 8, let alone 12, hours during the day without eating. Even a four-hour lag between meals leaves some people feeling shaky and down-right grumpy. Imagine what a 12-hour fast—from 7:00 p.m. to 7:00 a.m.—will do! When the alarm goes off the next morning, you—from your head to your toes—are basically running on fuel fumes. Sure you feel okay after a morning cup of coffee, mainly because alert hormones are at their peak in the morning and you've also had a bit of sleep. But it is counterfeit energy, since your brain and body are in serious need of a carb fix to restock those dwindling fuel stores. In fact, even if you eat a good lunch, you never regain the energy and brain power you would have had if you had taken five minutes to eat a decent breakfast.

The Natural High

Work with your natural rhythms by restocking fuel stores in the morning. Your body, mind and energy will repay you throughout the day.

Don't blame your dumb choice to skip breakfast on your brain. It tries its best to get you to eat from the moment you slap the snooze button. In its infinite wisdom, the body releases a brain chemical called neuro-peptide Y (NPY) at the dawn of each new day. NPY's job is to entice you to replenish carb stores. It does not care if you eat protein or fat. It is unconcerned about whether even one vitamin or mineral passes your lips. It's not even programmed to lead you in the direction of fiber. All it wants you to eat is carbs. NPY whispers to your unconscious to eat something starchy, much like the word *eat* flashed imperceptibly across a screen gets you thinking about that leftover piece of pie in the refrigerator. You do not feel the whoosh of NPY flooding your brain. You don't even label your hunger as a craving. It is more subtle than that. As the NPY travels through your brain, those German pancakes just start sounding really, really, *really* good.

It is no surprise then that most cultures around the world include a starch in their traditional breakfasts: In Japan it is rice, while in Paris it might be a croissant. A flat bread called injera is eaten in Ethiopia, while people in Ghana love sweetened bread and Costa Ricans eat pinto beans and rice. In the United States, it is pancakes, waffles, French toast, cereal, toast or doughnuts.

How you respond to NPY will have a subtle, but profound, effect on the rest of your day. Listen to your body, work with your natural impulses by adding a bagel along with your morning cup of brew and NPY has done its job—you restocked the glucose your body will need during morning hours. NPY is no longer needed, so levels drop to zero. Ignore this basic instinct by bolting out of the house with just the coffee, and you are likely to hit your own wall at some point during the day with foggy thinking, an irritable mood or low energy.

The Morning Train to Smartville

If you don't believe me, take a quick internal inventory. Right now, stop reading and check out how you feel. As you sit reading this sentence, for better or for worse, what you chose to eat or not eat for breakfast is affecting your ability to concentrate, analyze, remember, focus and even enjoy the moment. It's also affecting your mood and how alert you feel.

Alex went from breakfast skipper to breakfast advocate in her first year of college.

"I'd heard that breakfast was the most important meal of the day, but I really got the message when I came to college. If I don't eat breakfast before my morning class, I can barely make it to my break at noon. I get headachy and can't focus. But if I take a few minutes in the morning to eat something healthy, like peanut butter on toast with a piece of fruit, I sleep well, handle stress better and just feel more myself and energized. If I skip that meal and then don't eat regularly throughout the day, I become fatigued more quickly. I have to make time to eat, whether it's on the way to class or in the library. I am a total convert to the whole breakfast thing. I absolutely feel my best when I eat breakfast."

More often than not, the effects are subtle, but it's happening, whether you are attuned to your body or totally oblivious. So check yourself out. Are you feeling alert, vigorous, energetic, motivated, quick-thinking? Are you relaxed, calm, focused? Or are you feeling a tad bit irritated, grouchy or tense? How about sluggish? Slow? Sleepy? Sad? Now, what did you eat for breakfast? (If you can't remember, you are in bigger need of a morning makeover than I thought!)

I have a file drawer filled with research proving that people who eat breakfast are happier throughout the day (it has to be the right breakfast, of course, but we'll get to that later). They are upbeat with an even, consistent energy. They don't ride swells of energy highs and fatigue lows that breakfast skippers whine about around the doughnut box in the employees' lounge. They are more motivated and cheerful, less depressed and fatigued. Breakfast eaters are better problem solvers and are more alert. They also miss fewer days of school and work. Even math scores improve (and as far as I'm concerned, that's as close to a miracle as you can get!).

If you don't believe me, ask Lindsey, a public relations executive in Minneapolis, who says, "I didn't used to eat breakfast before work and I was always sluggish and distracted in the morning. When I became pregnant two years ago, I knew I had to start eating breakfast. What a difference that meal made. Ever since,

I almost always have breakfast, and I definitely notice that I am more alert and focused at work."

I can't promise that eating breakfast will guarantee you'll graduate magna cum laude from Harvard, go on to be a Rhodes scholar or win the Nobel Peace Prize, but you will enjoy life a whole lot more, lose a few pounds and maybe even get that raise.

Brand-New Carbs

The brain does not store energy like muscles do. Yesterday's pasta lunch or last night's popcorn snack does the brain little good the next morning. What it needs is brand-new glucose. The carbs in a good breakfast provide that—firing up the brain, providing just the type of fuel it likes best, so you think more clearly, are more creative, remember more, make fewer mistakes, score higher on intelligence tests and pay closer attention to details.

You also fret less. A study from Cardiff University in Wales where researchers investigated breakfast habits in 136 people between the ages of 23 and 60 found that those who took five minutes to eat a bowl of cereal in the morning had lower levels of the stress hormone cortisol.

Add a Meal, Lose an Inch

"I used to skip breakfast altogether—even skipped lunch, too, when I was in high school. It took me a while to figure out that bad habit was making me fat, fat, fat. Now I have a bowl of granola with fruit and nonfat milk four to five days a week. Surprise, surprise, I've lost all that weight and feel great, too!" says Linda, owner of a food-based company in the San Francisco Bay Area.

Interestingly, while many people admit they skip breakfast in hopes of losing weight, the very act of adding this meal cuts your risk of weight gain by half. It also is a key secret of people who have successfully maintained a big weight loss.

The National Weight Control Registry (NWCR), an ongoing study conducted at the University of Colorado and Brown University, has been researching the habits of thousands of people who have lost an average of 67 pounds (the range is from 30 to 300 pounds) and kept the weight off for more than seven years. One thing 90% of them do to keep the weight off is eat breakfast every day; only 4% are complete breakfast skippers. In contrast, another study from Massachusetts Medical School in Worcester found that breakfast skippers were a whopping 450% more likely to be obese than regular breakfast eaters. Wow. Those skinnier people must be onto something!

First, breakfast perks up your metabolism so you burn about 150 calories more than if you skipped this meal. That might not sound like much, but it is the calorie equivalent of a small bag of chips or three Oreo cookies. Burn 150 extra calories every day (or give up the chips and cookies) and over the course of a year that equates to a 15-pound weight loss. Second, choose the right mix of foods at breakfast and you hush hunger pangs for hours.

Study after study shows that people who eat healthy breakfasts are less likely to impulse snack later in the day. They also are satisfied on fewer calories at lunch and even dinner. A breakfast rich in three ingredients—water, protein and fiber—is what leads to the biggest weight loss. In fact, one study found that a high-fiber, low-fat breakfast satisfied people for up to six hours, or two hours longer than a low-fiber breakfast.

What's so magical about these three ingredients? Water incorporated into food, such as cooked oatmeal, fills you up on few calories. Protein helps balance blood sugar and keeps you full longer. Most important is the fiber, which slows digestion and lowers a food's glycemic index (GI), a measurement of how fast and how dramatically food raises blood sugar levels. Low-GI foods give you a nice, gentle boost in blood sugar, while high-GI foods dump sugar into your blood faster than a flood rushing downhill. As a result, low-GI foods improve your chances of avoiding diabetes and dropping pounds. Low-GI foods, such as oatmeal, are the best at weight management and improving memory and job or school performance, while keeping your brain sharp and focused. Fiber-rich foods also might stimulate a hormone that keeps you feeling full longer. (More on the glycemic index in Chapter 3.)

The Big Seven for Weight Loss

The top seven most important habits of successful dieting include

- Get eight hours of sleep every night.
- Eat breakfast!
- Walk briskly for at least 60 minutes a day (see Chapter 11).
- Write down what you eat.
- Weigh yourself frequently.
- Get support from family, a peer group, a 12-step program, friends, neighbors, coworkers.
- Never, never, never give up!

Compared to people who fill up on refined grains, happy, fit people consume at least three fiber-packed whole grains a day, which explains why they have a much lower body mass index (BMI), a measurement of body weight to height with low BMIs reflecting leaner bodies. Fiber-rich and/or water-packed foods, such as oatmeal, brown rice pudding, a fruit smoothie or whole-grain cereal, also typically are low calorie, so you fill up without filling out.

Remember NPY, the brain chemical that wants you to eat carbs? Well, it only stops sending the message if you follow its instructions. Ignore the memo and the messenger sticks around. It digs in, camps out and marshals its forces. Jammed in high gear, NPY levels stay elevated well into the middle of the day, whispering and then screaming for carbs. This might explain why people who skip breakfast tend to overeat—and eat all the wrong carb-rich stuff from midafternoon until bedtime. It also might partially explain why potato chips are the number one snack food for breakfast skippers!

Bowled Over

Breakfast eaters typically have overall diets that are richer in brain-tickling, mood-elevating goodies like vitamins (such as folate and vitamins C and D), minerals (such as iron, zinc, calcium and magnesium), fiber, antioxidant-packed phytonutrients and healthy fats, and a whole lot less dumbing-down naughties like saturated fats, cholesterol, trans fats and sugar.

No big surprise here. Thanks to a freak of nature, people are more likely to choose more nutritious foods in the morning than at any other time of the day. Even if it is Cap'n Crunch, a bowl of cereal is the most nutritious meal of the day for many people. Not just because it is a low-fat grain, but also because of the company it keeps, which provides a nutritional edge that you never make up for elsewhere.

Cereal with its accompaniments is one of many food groupings, called a "food cluster." You know them by sight. For example,

The fast-food cluster:
Hamburger, fries and soft drink

The movie cluster:
Popcorn, candy bar and soft drink

The baseball cluster:
Hot dog, peanuts and beer

The breakfast cluster:
Whole-grain cereal, nonfat milk and fruit

Of all those choices, the cereal cluster is the only one that's good for you, loaded with calcium and protein. And since only a weirdo would heap those flakes with artery-clogging bacon and cheese, the typical toppings of blueberries or a sliced banana add extra vitamin C, antioxidants and fiber—and no fat. No wonder a study found that women who fill up on the breakfast cluster of cereal, milk and fruit consume fewer calories at lunch and have overall diets lower in fat. They also are more alert.

Red Alert! Asleep at the Wheel Breakfasts

Not all breakfasts are created equal. Whether at a restaurant, in the freezer case at the grocery store or in recipe books and magazines at home, anything with eggs, cheese, cream cheese or butter and/or ham, sausage or bacon is likely to be a breakfast nightmare. Greasy breakfasts high in fat, sodium and calories do just the opposite of those high-fiber, low-fat bowls of cereal. For example, choose a Red Baron Mini Scramble with Ham from the freezer case and 40% of the 400 calories will be coming from fat, yet with only a measly 1 gram of fiber. More than 42% of the calories in a Hot Pockets Bacon, Egg & Cheese comes from fat, while almost 90% of the calories in an Armour Beef Brown & Serve sausage is grease. (If you can't live without some meat at breakfast, try one or two Morningstar Farms vegetarian sausages, which have half the calories and a fraction of the fat of Brown & Serve sausages.) Foods like these leave you feeling sluggish because that glut of fat entering the bloodstream blocks oxygen flow to the brain. Like a clogged drain, your brain is deprived of a free-flowing blood supply. It is no surprise that these meals leave you unable to think straight and more prone to daydream or nap than to eagerly dive into a project at work or an exam at school.

The very worst carb choices for breakfast include the gooey carbs, like a Danish, doughnut, toaster pastries or cinnamon roll, since they are loaded with sugar, refined grains, sodium and fat and are pathetically low on fiber, protein, phytonutrients and every vitamin or mineral you can name.

These choices wreak havoc with blood sugar levels down the morning road, leaving you more prepared for a siesta than a board meeting—not to mention the long-term damage to your heart and waistline (see "Blood Sugar Boogie: The Glycemic Index" in Chapter 3). What NPY wants, what your brain and body need and what you should be looking for is the type of quality breakfast that happy, fit people eat.

Clean Up Your Breakfast Act

Instead of....	Have....
Cinnamon Chip Scone at Starbucks (510 calories, 23 grams fat)	1 cup cinnamon-flavored whole-grain cereal, nonfat milk, ½ banana. (260 calories, 1 gram fat)
Loaded Breakfast Burrito at Hardee's (780 calories, 51 grams fat)	A Mission Life Balance tortilla filled with 2 scrambled egg whites, 1 oz Cabot Vermont 50% Reduced Fat Cheese, ¼ cup cilantro, ½ tomato sliced, 2 tablespoons salsa. Serve with 1 cup low-fat milk. (302 calories, 5 grams fat)
Sausage, Egg & Cheese Croissant at Dunkin' Donuts (650 calories, 45 grams fat)	Whole-wheat English muffin topped with 1 scrambled egg white, 2 oz veggie sausage patty, 1 large tomato slice and 1 oz low-fat cheese, broiled. Serve with 1 cup low-fat milk and 1 cup fresh strawberries. (473 calories, 7.6 grams fat)

Sesame Bagel with Cream Cheese at Einstein Bros. (450 calories, 12 grams fat)	Whole-wheat bagel topped with fat-free cream cheese with strawberry jam. Serve with 1 cup low-fat milk and 1 cup cantaloupe. (449 calories, 2 grams fat)
Delux Warm Cinnamon Roll at McDonald's (590 calories, 24 grams fat)	1 slice toasted 100% whole-wheat bread topped with 1 teaspoon butter and cinnamon sugar. Serve with 1 cup low-fat milk and 1 cup mango slices. (315 calories, 6 grams fat)
Honey Raisin Bran Muffin at Dunkin' Donuts (480 calories, 15 grams fat)	1 small low-fat bran muffin served with 1 cup warm low-fat milk flavored with vanilla extract and Splenda, and 1 orange sectioned and sprinkled with crystalline ginger. (396 calories, 11 grams fat)

The 1-2-3 Rule

If you haven't eaten breakfast since the days when Mom packed your lunch, you probably feel a bit lost at this point. You know you need to eat something in the morning, but what? It's not just *when* you eat, but *what* you choose that will make all the difference in your mood and your waistline. Choose the right mix of foods and you will reap all the energizing benefits that happy, fit people experience every day. Skip the meal or wolf down a Pop-Tart and coffee and you'll be sliding into grumpville by afternoon.

Of course, time is of the essence. Your morning routine probably looks more like a mob stampede from a burning building than a calm, zen-filled meditation. In the afterdawn, mad-dash chaos packed with making lunches, grabbing clothes out of the dryer, fighting over the shower, feeding the dog or the iguana, looking for that other earring, brushing your teeth and multitasking everything (ever blow-dried your hair while sitting on the toilet?), fixing a nutritious breakfast might be just the last straw that breaks your emotional camel's back.

I don't want to hear any whining. Happy, fit people are just as busy as you are. Their mornings are seldom perfect. They juggle the same morning mess, they oversleep, they wake up on the wrong side of the bed, their kids refuse to get up, the suit they needed is rumpled and their panty hose have runs in them, too. But they eat breakfast anyway. How do they do it? They follow the 1-2-3 Rule.

Excuses, Excuses, Excuses

Many people are their own worst enemies when it comes to making diet changes or losing weight. They want to be healthier, have more energy, think faster, look younger and be thinner, but they give up the power to make those changes by putting the blame for not reaching those goals on something or someone else. The truth is, there is a solution to every single excuse. So let's bust a few right now:

I would eat breakfast, but...

1. I don't have time. Too busy to eat breakfast? Actually, you are too busy *not to* is more like it! Breakfast is the quickest meal to get on the table. It only takes five minutes to fix and eat a nutritious breakfast! Yet that time investment will pay off a thousandfold throughout the day. You'll get more done, think faster, have more energy and enjoy yourself more when there is quality fuel firing the engines. Get up five minutes earlier, fix a smoothie the night before, bring breakfast with you or have a "desk fast" meal once you get to work. (Besides, how many times have I heard a person say she had no time to eat breakfast, but then complain about the line at Starbucks? If you have no time at home, what are you doing at the coffee shop?!)

2. I'm not hungry in the morning. You should be hungry. It has been 8 to 12 hours since you last ate. Any other time of the day, that lengthy fast would leave you ravenous. My guess is you used to be hungry but ignored the signals and your body stopped sending them. Start eating a light breakfast, such as a piece of whole-wheat toast topped with peanut butter and a glass of tomato juice. Within two weeks, you will reprogram your tastebuds and appetite clock to expect a little "something" in the morning.

3. I don't like breakfast foods. Who says you have to eat cereal or pancakes or any typical breakfast food in the morning? As long as your meal meets the 1-2-3 Rule, you can have anything you want, such as pizza topped with vegetables, a turkey sandwich piled high with lettuce on whole wheat, cold macaroni and cheese with an orange, vegetable soup and a PBJ sandwich, or chili with cornbread and a fruit salad.

4. I'm hungry all day if I eat breakfast. It's not the breakfast, silly! Increased hunger is caused not by breakfast, but more likely by the foods you choose. Sugary foods eaten alone, whether they are sugar-coated cereals, doughnuts or fruit, don't stick with you and leave you hungry within an hour or so. Whitney, a public relations executive in San Francisco, found that the 1-2-3 Rule worked best for her;

"I definitely notice changes in the way I feel the entire day depending on what I eat for breakfast. A light breakfast of toast or fruit leaves me hungry, shaky and nervous by noon. But if I add plain Greek low-fat yogurt and walnuts to the mix, it makes a huge difference. I'm not hungry for lunch nearly so early and my blood sugar is kept in check the entire day."

5. I exercise in the morning, so I can't eat. Even a small snack five minutes beforehand is better than nothing and can enhance performance. However, timing is important. Plan to snack one to two hours before your workout to enhance your performance without upsetting your stomach. Liquids digest faster than solids, so an 8-ounce fruit and yogurt smoothie or a glass of Instant Breakfast made with nonfat milk or soy milk might be your best bet if you snack within the hour before a run or any vigorous or bouncy sport. Have a bigger meal but allow more time—up to four hours—before jumping into a heavy-duty workout, to ensure food has emptied from the stomach and is at least partially digested. Of course, if that hefty workout is at 6:00 a.m., it's not likely you'll get up at 4:00 a.m. to eat. In this case, have something light, such as a few graham crackers, as you head out the door for that 6-mile run. Then finish your breakfast when you get done.

So what is this magical 1-2-3 Rule? It is a formula that mixes and matches foods for a healthy breakfast packed with the mood-boosting, energizing nutrients discussed in Chapter 7. You don't need to stock unrecognizable foods in your pantry, take a course in nutrition or even know how to cook to put this formula into practice. Best of all, the 1-2-3 breakfast takes five minutes or less to fix *and* eat. Here is all you need to kick-start an energizing day. Combine

1. One to three servings of a quality, high-fiber carbohydrate

2. Two servings of fruits (or vegetables)

3. One protein

Let's look at this 1-2-3 Rule in more detail.

Number One in the 1-2-3 Breakfast: One to Three Servings of Quality, High-Fiber Carbs

High-quality carbs supply the glucose your brain and body need to restock fuel stores and keep blood sugar levels even throughout the morning. They satisfy NPY levels, so you won't pig out later in the day. The fiber fills you up on fewer calories and will stick with you so you are satisfied throughout the morning and less likely to nibble those chocolate Kisses off a coworker's desk or rummage through the fridge or your kids' old Halloween candy at home. In fact, one study found that women had a 49% lower risk of gaining weight when they included more whole grains and less refined grains in their diets.

One serving of a high-quality, high-fiber choice includes, but is not limited to:

- 1 to 2 ounces of ready-to-eat, 100% whole-grain cereal (such as Kashi Autumn Wheat, Food for Life's Ezekial 4:9 Original, Nature's Path Organic Heritage O's, Shredded Wheat, or Grape-Nuts). Then take it to the nutritional top by sprinkling it with some super mood food, like toasted wheat germ, which is chock full of vitamin E, B vitamins, trace minerals and choline, an important memory-enhancing nutrient.

- 1 slice 100% whole-wheat bread, ½ whole-wheat bagel or English muffin, 1 whole-wheat flour tortilla or low-fat whole-wheat scone
- 1 small (2 ounces) low-fat muffin, preferably whole wheat, bran or carrot
- A slice of cornbread
- ½ cup cooked whole-grain hot cereal, such as oatmeal, multigrain cereal, brown rice, polenta or barley
- 1 4" pancake, whole-wheat waffle or French toast. To make your favorite morning carb more nutritious; add toasted wheat germ to your pancake or waffle batters and switch to whole-wheat bread for the French toast.
- Peek into the freezer case at your local grocery store. You will find plenty of frozen breakfasts that deliver nutrition and taste in minutes. Look for options that contain no more than 300 calories, 1 to 2 grams saturated fat, 0 trans fats, and 480 milligrams sodium, and at least 2 grams fiber per serving.

You don't want to romp through the morning filled with Honey Bunches of Junk or Cocoa Fluffs. There are more than 400 ready-to-eat cereals on grocery shelves, most of which try to trick you into thinking a chocolate-covered, overly sweet cereal is actually good for you. Don't be fooled by brands that say "Made with whole grain" or "a good source of whole grain." Instead

1. Flip the box over and check out the nutritional panel. A rule of thumb is that the higher the sugar, the lower the fiber. Remember the number 5. You want only cereals with

- no more than about 5 grams of sugar and
- 5 or more grams of fiber

2. Then read the ingredients list. The fewer ingredients and the more of them you recognize and can pronounce, the better. Also, whole grains, such as whole wheat, oats, rye, barley or millet, should be the only grain—or at least the first grains. Your best bet is to look for cereals that say "100% whole grain." That guarantees a quality, high-fiber grain. Another rule of thumb is the less refined the grains in a cereal or bread are, the lower its sodium content. For example, old-fashioned oats have no sodium, while instant oats have 260 milligrams of sodium for every half cup cooked.

3. The less processed, the more filling a cereal will be and the longer it will "stick with you" through the morning. That's because it takes the body longer to break down the fibrous, unprocessed grains, so your tummy is busy digesting and not thinking about the next meal. Unprocessed grains also have low-GI scores, so they provide a nice, even blood sugar level rather than the blood sugar roller-coaster ride you get from refined grains. Both barley and oats contain a type of fiber called beta-glucan that digests slowly and keeps you feeling full the longest. In short,

> Irish oat groats > Quaker Old-Fashioned Oats > Quaker Simple Harvest Hot Cereal > Quaker Instant Oatmeal > Quaker Apples & Cinnamon Instant Oatmeal

Are you a cereal monogamist? Do you eat the same bowl of flakes day in and day out, every morning and sometimes for dinner, too? Come on, you need to spice up your life a bit! Add some adventure to your morning with these tips:

Mix it up. Blend two to three cereals together, such as Shredded Wheat and Fiber One Honey Clusters, then top with walnuts and raisins. This is also a good way to dilute the calories in a high-fat cereal, such as granola, or a high-sugar cereal, such as Cranberry Crunch, by sprinkling them on top of a lower fat or more nutritious cereal, like Ezekiel or Weetabix.

Make it taste like pie. Add canned pumpkin and pumpkin spices to oatmeal. Or cook oatmeal in milk flavored with almond extract and sprinkle slivered almonds on top.

Change the texture. Add Grape-Nuts, trail mix, peach chunks or banana slices to hot or cold cereal.

Number Two in the 1-2-3 Breakfast: Two Servings of Fruits and Vegetables

Do not eat cereal naked! No, I don't mean put on your sweats before you eat. I mean the cereal itself, silly. Top it with brain-protecting superfoods, such as berries, dried plums, figs or banana slices, or mix apple chunks, dried tart cherries or mango bits into it. These super mood foods give your brain the antioxidants it needs to defend itself throughout the morning hours from oxygen fragments, called free radicals or oxidants, that damage cell membranes and lead to muddled minds. Grab colorful fruits and vegetables, since the antioxidants are in the pigment (that means "color")—the more pigment, the more antioxidants. Take advantage of tons of research showing that some fruits and vegetables really boost brain power, from blueberries to dried plums.

When you think color, think berries, cherries, tomatoes and oranges. Grab a kiwi, a mango, a half papaya or a banana. Drink carrot juice, tomato juice or prune juice. To make your favorite morning 1-2-3 breakfast more nutritious, skip the syrup and instead pile fresh fruit on top of waffles, French toast or pancakes. You can have two different fruits and vegetables, or just double a serving

What is a serving? It isn't the three blueberries in a Starbucks muffin, the hint of strawberry in that crunch cereal or even the smattering of raisins in a bowl of Raisin Bran. One serving is:

- *6 ounces 100% fruit or vegetable juice.* Avoid all juices made with "pure grape, pear or apple juice concentrate," since these "all natural" fruit beverages are just plain old sugar water. Instead, choose 100% orange juice, grapefruit juice, orange-pineapple juice or tomato juice. Or fresh squeeze your own juices if you have time.
- *One small fruit,* such as a plum, pear, apple, banana, orange, tangerine, grapefruit, kiwi or peach. Or half a cantaloupe, other melon or papaya.
- *½ cup fruit*—fresh, frozen or canned in its own juice
- *2 tablespoons dried fruit,* such as dried tart cherries, apricots, prunes or currants
- *One medium tomato,* sliced
- *½ cup steamed mixed vegetables* added to an omelet or wrap

What about hash browns or any frozen fried potato? I dare you to find a brand that has less than 3 grams of fat for every 100 calories *and* contains no hydrogenated vegetable oil, which is a prime source of trans fats, another type of fat known to increase heart disease and possibly dampen mood. If you can find a brand that meets this criteria, and you don't add any additional fat in preparation, then these are okay to include once in a while. But they certainly are no substitute for orange juice, cantaloupe or tomato slices or any richly colored fruit or vegetable.

Number Three in the 1-2-3 Breakfast: One Serving of a Protein-Rich Food

This part of the 1-2-3 Rule provides staying power. Assuming you make the right choice, protein-rich foods slow digestion. While an all-carb breakfast can leave you searching for a snack within an hour or two, add some protein to that meal and you can get on with your life without thinking about food for at least four hours. Remember, the protein-rich milk or soy milk on your cereal does you no good poured down the drain. Besides, many of those vitamins and minerals in the fortified cereals dissolve into the milk, so tip the bowl and drink it up when the cereal is gone or you are wasting a lot of nutrition! (Added tip: To make your favorite 1-2-3 breakfast more nutritious, read labels and choose only breakfast meats—sausage, ham, bacon, etc.—that contain no more than 3 grams total fat and 1 gram saturated fat for every 100 calories.)

Limited evidence also suggests that the calcium in super mood foods, like milk and yogurt, help you burn fat and store less of it, while preserving muscles. For every extra glass of milk, a person can expect to lose between two and six pounds of body fat. (See Chapter 5 on the superfoods.) So, it's a one-two-three punch for mood and waist management. Your protein choices include

- *Dairy:* Fat-free or low-fat milk or yogurt (1 cup), cottage cheese (2 cups), cheese (1 ounce) or ricotta cheese (2 ounces)
- *Soy:* Plain, vanilla or light soy milk (1 cup)
- *Meat:* A thin slice of meat, such as turkey, chicken, beef (1 to 3 ounces)
- *Legumes:* Cooked dried beans and peas, such as peanut or almond butter (2 tablespoons), breakfast beans (1 cup) or tofu (3 to 4 ounces). Breakfast is a perfect time to load up on these super mood foods, which are rich in phytochemicals called sterols, stanols and phytoestrogens that lower blood cholesterol and cancer risk.
- *Eggs:* ¼ to ½ cup egg substitute, 1 whole egg or 2 egg whites

The 1-Minute Breakfast

You overslept and now there isn't even time for a five-minute glance at the kitchen. You still can make it to work and fuel your brain for a happy day by making breakfast irresistibly convenient. These grab-and-go "Purseables" or "Briefcase-ables" will do on those days that start like a gunshot at a 10-K race.

- A carton of nonfat milk, a banana and an energy bar that has at least 7 grams protein, less than 8 grams sugar and more than 3 grams fiber, such as Kashi's TLC Crunchy or Chewy bars

- 2 low-fat cheese sticks, a mini whole-wheat bagel and an orange. Boost brain power by adding a cup of green tea, too

- A hard-boiled egg, a slice of 100% whole-wheat bread and a 6-ounce can of tomato juice

- A McDonald's Fruit 'n' Yogurt Parfait with Granola, along with a piece of fruit from home

- A small bran muffin, Rachel's yogurt and an 8-ounce carton of calcium- and vitamin D–fortified OJ

- Get a six-pack of portable 8-ounce milks (fat-free or low-fat), label them and put them in the office fridge for the week. Keep single-serve boxes of whole-grain cereals, oranges and other fruits that keep in your desk. When you get to the office, prepare your own "desk-fest"—cereal and milk. Not only is it nutritious, but it's less expensive than getting a daily doughnut at the shop down the street!

- Make your breakfast the night before. Before you go to bed, place ½ cup old-fashioned oats, 2 tablespoons chopped dried fruit, 1 tablespoon brown sugar and a dash of cinnamon and almond extract in a preheated, wide-mouth thermos. Add 1 cup of steamed fat-free or low-fat milk or soy milk and close tightly. In the morning, just open the thermos, sprinkle with 2 teaspoons of slivered almonds, and you have a warm, delicious breakfast waiting for you!

- The night before, place your favorite smoothie ingredients in a blender and place in the fridge. It will take only 20 seconds in the morning to whip up breakfast.

Start Right, End Strong

You wouldn't dream of not recharging your cell phone when anticipating an important phone call, just as you'd look pretty stupid taking off on a cross-country road trip without filling up the car with gas. Treat your body with the same respect and kindness as you prepare for your day. Every time you put something into your mouth, you are choosing whether or not to care for yourself. Make sure to start the day right and work with your natural body rhythms, and you'll be on your way to being that happy, fit person you've always dreamed you could be.

Two Weeks of Instant Breakfasts

Putting the 1-2-3 Rule into practice is as simple as

1. Mix a bowl of whole-grain cereal, low-fat milk or soy milk and fruit.

2. Fill a corn tortilla with scrambled Gold Circle Farm eggs and salsa. Serve with OJ.

3. Cook instant oatmeal or multigrain cereal in milk in the microwave, top with walnuts and brown sugar, and serve with apricot nectar or fresh fruit.

4. Stuff scrambled eggs or egg substitute, chopped tomatoes and cilantro in whole-wheat pita bread. Serve with nonfat milk and fresh fruit.

5. Add fresh peach slices, dried cranberries, almonds and whole-grain cereal to nonfat yogurt.

6. Serve apple-cinnamon yogurt, a slice of toasted raisin bread topped with peanut butter and nectarine slices.

7. Top a whole-wheat English muffin with thick slices of tomato and a thin slice of low-fat cheese. Broil. Serve with pineapple juice.

8. Top a toasted whole-grain frozen waffle with fat-free sour cream and blueberries. Serve with milk.

9. Top a toasted half whole-wheat bagel with lox and fat-free cream cheese, red onion and sprouts. Serve with milk or OJ.

10. Enjoy a Lean Pockets Bacon, Egg & Cheese with a glass of OJ.

11. Mix equal parts peanut butter, toasted wheat germ and honey. Spread on 100% whole-wheat bread. Serve with fresh fruit and milk.

12. Fill a half cantaloupe with nonfat lemon yogurt and sprinkle with granola.

13. Serve a Morningstar Farms Breakfast Sandwich with Cheese and a sliced pear.

14. Top two slices of rye bread with two slices Canadian bacon and one medium tomato, sliced. Serve with OJ,

SECRET 3:
CHOOSE QUALITY CARBS

The Promise

In one week of making this change, you will:

- feel full on fewer calories
- notice an improvement in energy throughout the day

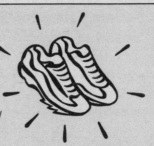

In one month, you will:

- notice an improvement in mood
- experience more energy (and more even energy) throughout the day
- feel less stressed
- sleep better
- think more clearly
- be less likely to binge on junk food

In one year, you will:

- lose weight

Nowhere is the link between food, mood and waist-line more obvious than with carbs. Take Colleen, for example, a legal secretary in La Mesa, California, who for years fought a battle between the angel of good diet intentions on one shoulder and the devil of carb treats on the other.

She came to me after her most recent failed dieting attempt, which had left her 5 pounds heavier. "I'm a tried-and-true carb addict, especially when I'm under pressure. I've been the slave of pretzels, muffins and potato chips for years," she confessed, looking apologetically at me, the diet priest, as if waiting to be absolved of her diet sins.

Colleen gained 7 pounds her freshman year of college, soothing stress with muffins and other carb-rich junk from the dorm cafeteria.

The habit stuck and escalated once she entered the workforce. "One of the attorneys in my office is a real perfection freak. If I forget to dot an *i* or if I staple the papers incorrectly, let me tell you, I hear about it big-time. That pressure really stresses me out!" She tried bringing baby carrots and string cheese to work to curb hunger pangs, but typically ended up across the street agonizing between the Glazin' Raisin Pretzel and the Sesame Pretzel at Auntie Anne's.

Colleen's latest weight-loss failure had been a low-carb diet. "I thought going cold turkey on my weakness for pretzels and chips might do the trick," she groaned. But it backfired. She was carb-free for three weeks and lost 12 pounds, but then a particularly bad day at work left her miserable. With shoulders rock-hard tense and a raging headache, the carb cravings came back with a vengeance. "It felt like Mount Saint Helens about to explode. I could no more stop the urge to eat a cookie than stop the eruption. I ate an entire bag of Doritos in the car before I even got home." She showed up at my office three weeks later.

Why Carbs Are a Natural High

If, like Colleen, you head for the chips, muffins, pretzels, oatmeal, bread, pasta or any other carbohydrate-rich food when feeling tense, nervous, stressed out, grumpy or tired, more than likely it is a serotonin fix you are after.

You have probably heard of serotonin. It is the nerve chemical, or neurotransmitter, that is switched on by some of America's favorite antidepressant medications, from Celexa and Cymbalta to Prozac and Paxil. Of course, our bodies naturally make serotonin, but sometimes not enough. This nerve chemical is a major force in mood and appetite. It turns on and off cravings for sweets and starches, helps regulate mood, controls pain tolerance, affects thinking and memory and even determines whether we sleep well. Boost serotonin levels, either naturally or with medication, and your cravings subside, you are more relaxed and happier and you sleep more soundly. High serotonin levels have even calmed people prone to violence, increased pain tolerance so people handle the dentist's drill with less novocaine and soothed the melancholy jags of both premenstrual syndrome (PMS) and the winter blues.

In contrast, when serotonin takes a nosedive, so does your mood and ability to think straight, while you are likely to pig out on carbs and sleep fitfully. You also are more likely to lose your cool during stress. Not a pretty picture, but one that many people can relate to. You've probably guessed it already—happy, fit people know how to keep their serotonin levels high, or at least not low.

The Natural High

Work with your cravings and in tune with serotonin and you sidestep many of the problems associated with problem eating, fatigue, premenstrual syndrome (PMS), seasonal affective disorder (SAD) and depression.

No other neurotransmitter is as sensitive to diet choices as is serotonin. This neurotransmitter is manufactured in the brain from an amino acid called tryptophan, which is found in protein-rich foods, such as turkey, milk, eggs, meat, nuts and beans. You may have heard that the reason why turkey at Thanksgiving or a warm glass of milk at night before bed makes you sleepy is because these foods are rich in tryptophan, so they raise serotonin levels. Not true! Protein-rich foods are high in the building block for serotonin, but eating them actually deadlocks serotonin. Only carbs raise serotonin in the brain and soothe both your mood funk and your cravings. (Actually, one other nutrient raises serotonin—the omega-3 fat DHA—but I'll get to that in Chapter 6.)

The reason why pretzels, but not turkey, could boost Colleen's serotonin is a bit tricky, so put on your thinking cap.

Tryptophan is a large amino acid that competes with other amino acids, such as tyrosine, to get through the blood-brain barrier (the series of membranes, enzymes and blood vessels that separate the brain from the body). When you eat a protein-rich meal, you flood the blood with both tryptophan and the other 20+ "competing amino acids," creating a free-for-all where they all fight for entry into the brain. Think of it as the line at the movie theater to see Harry Potter. If you are the only one buying a ticket, there is no wait and you get first-choice seating inside. But if 100 people got there before you, it will be a long wait, the tickets may be sold out by the time you reach the head of the line, or you will end up at the back of the theater sitting behind a guy the size of a linebacker.

The same goes for tryptophan. A protein-rich food supplies tons of competition, which means tryptophan loses—only small amounts make it through the blood-brain barrier, little serotonin is made, and you miss out on the needed mood boost.

While turkey or any other protein-rich food won't give you a serotonin high, carbs will. Little did Colleen know that a starchy food like pretzels was exactly what she needed to feel better, and, in fact, those cravings were an unconscious attempt to self-medicate. Once starch is digested, a flood of carbs enter the blood, which triggers the release of insulin, a hormone from the pancreas. Insulin returns blood sugar levels to normal and ushers many amino acids (either from the meal or just floating in the blood) into the tissues. But insulin ignores tryptophan, leaving it behind in the blood. With the competing amino acids gone, tryptophan is the only one standing in line at the blood-brain barrier. It has a straight, unhindered shot into the brain. In short,

1. The more tryptophan that makes it across the barrier, the higher the concentration in the brain.
2. The higher the concentration of tryptophan in the brain, the more serotonin is made.
3. The higher your serotonin levels, the happier you are.

Serotonin is the classic chicken-and-egg scenario. This nerve chemical is dependent on what you eat, while what you choose to eat, in part, is dictated by the level of serotonin. When serotonin levels are low, you crave carbohydrates, such as sweets or starches, which are the very foods that raise brain levels of both tryptophan and serotonin and turn off the cravings. In short, cravers unconsciously turn to desserts, doughnuts and other pastries, pasta, cereals, muffins, scones or breads to relieve dwindling energy levels, grumpiness and depression brought on by low serotonin levels. The snack works—it raises serotonin levels, curbs cravings and boosts the craver's mood. Once serotonin levels are high, the carb craving subsides.

Why Low-Carb Diets Don't Work

The link between carbs and mood explains why carbohydrate-cravers like Colleen can't live forever on low-carb diets. These diets prevent the brain from making enough serotonin, which leaves the dieter fatigued, grumpy, stressed and miserable. Sure, they start the diet with gusto, energized and hopeful that this time the weight will drop off for good. They lose some pounds, but after a few weeks of existing on serotonin fumes, they emotionally cave.

That is what happened to Colleen. After three weeks on a low-carb diet, she felt lousy, antsy and depressed. All it took was one stressful day (though it could have been a change in routine, such as a trip or altered work schedule), and—oops!—back to the old eating habits with a vengeance. As I told Colleen, "If you want to lose weight, you need to feel good. And to feel good, you need to work with your serotonin levels. You need to get this clear—it is not only possible to feel great while dieting, it is essential to success!"

Happy, fit carb cravers know all about this. They choose the right carbs in the right amounts to work in tune with their bodies to get a natural high, raising serotonin and sidestepping many of the problems associated with fad diets and stress, as well as PMS, seasonal affective disorder (SAD) and depression. They know if they don't work with serotonin—that is, if they snack on too much of the wrong stuff, follow silly low-carb diets or skip meals—they will pay for it emotionally and weight-wise.

How Do I Know It Is Serotonin?

Good question. While there is no handy test for measuring your serotonin levels, you can figure it out with a little self-assessing and a bit of trial and error.

First, ask yourself the question I asked Colleen: Do you turn to carbs when you are...

- bored?
- tired?
- need to relax?
- lonely?
- irritated or grumpy?
- trying to quit smoking or alcohol?
- feeling fidgety or restless?
- unable to concentrate?
- impatient?

- edgy?
- angry or mad?
- tense?
- depressed, sad, blue or gloomy?
- stressed or overwhelmed?

- disappointed in yourself?
- menopausal? (for women only)
- in the 10 to 14 days before your period? (for women only)

The more often you answered "yes" to the above questions, the more likely you are seeking a serotonin fix.

Second, when you are feeling any of the above emotions, can you put your finger on a specific reason why? Are you dead tired because you were up all night studying for a final exam, completing a project for work or soothing a cranky newborn? Are you super-stressed about meeting a deadline or concerned about your teenager? Are you worried or down because your relationship is in trouble or a promotion at work passed you by? Are you stressed out because your bills add up to more than your bank account? Are you facing a life-threatening disease? If not and there is no other obvious reason, or if your reason is just a flimsy excuse ("I'm getting older," "I was born grumpy") then it is even more likely that the problem is your diet. Of course, even if there is a justifiable reason why you feel blue, making a few diet changes for the better always, always, *always* helps.

Third, do you eat more from your stomach or from your head? If you are an experienced dieter, jumping on every fad that comes along from food combining to low-carb, you may have lost the connection to what real hunger feels like. Dieting numbs the hunger response, so you can lose the ability to know when you are hungry or full. Fad diets tell you what and when to eat, so you learn to eat according to outside rules, rather than inside hunger.

Repeat dieters also are more likely to interpret all troubling feelings as hunger. It's an understandable trade-off. Probably nothing else in life is as firmly rooted in security as is food. As babies, the most powerful comforter when we are upset is food, so it makes sense that we would continue to turn to that symbol of comfort as adults. Grabbing a carb-rich muffin is like trying to return to that security, that home, that safe place. So, food becomes a tranquilizer when we're anxious and a mood elevator when we're depressed. It fills us up when we're emotionally starved, comforts us when we're lonely and entertains us when we're bored. When we eat from our head or heart, rather than stomach, it is easy to be thinking about food all day long.

Unfortunately, turning to food for something other than physical nourishment only works in the short-term and ends up trading one problem (feeling cranky or mad) for another (fatigue or more belly fat). So, ask yourself,

"Do I turn to (fill in this blank, i.e., doughnuts, muffins, toaster pastries) when I am truly hungry, or is it more of a head or heart thing? Do I listen to my body, eating most often because I am physically hungry, with symptoms such as an empty feeling in your stomach, lightheadedness or my stomach growling? Or do I eat because the food is there, someone else is eating, I'm lonely or sad or bored or just because the food looks good?"

If you still aren't sure whether it's your stomach or your head that entices you to eat, then ponder the following scenarios. If any of these sound familiar, it is a good sign that serotonin, in concert with emotions, is at the helm of your food choices.

- You plan to have a skinny latte at the coffee shop but see the cranberry walnut scone and decide to have that, too.
- At the party, you sample more than you need from the buffet table because it all looks so good.
- While walking by the cinnamon roll shop at the mall, your friend suggests you share a roll; even though you are not hungry, you say yes.
- When home alone on a Friday night, your date is food.
- You grab a doughnut in the employees' lounge because someone said they were tasty.

When Cravings Go Bad

At one time or another, most of us have turned to food for solace, comfort or relaxation. In most cases, the indulgence is harmless and comforting. However, some people, in an effort to soothe a funky mood (by kick-starting serotonin levels), choose foods that unknowingly make them feel worse and set up a vicious cycle of feeling bad and overeating. This is particularly true for anyone battling seasonal affective disorder, depression in general, repeat dieters or women with PMS. Most of the time, these people also battle cravings and weight gain.

Consciously or unconsciously, happy, fit people work with serotonin to at least improve, if not solve, these doldrums. The alternative leads to real problems. When people don't work with their body's natural balance, when they eat the wrong stuff, at the wrong times, in the wrong amounts, they only make matters worse. The temporary false "high" from a carb binge is followed by a worse "low," leaving only one option—to reach, once again, for another bad-carb fix, which creates a vicious cycle leading to weight gain and self-loathing.

The Quality Carb Solution

As happy, fit people know, when you make the right food choices, the payoff is huge! Serotonin levels rise twofold with the right foods. That means a pleasant improvement in your night life, since it can cut in half the time that it takes to fall asleep and help you sleep longer and sounder. Imagine waking up refreshed, eager for a new day! If you don't believe me, listen to the researchers at the University of Sydney. Their study found that insomniacs fell asleep the fastest after eating a light, all-carb snack an hour before bedtime. If zzzs elude you, then a carb-rich bedtime snack is your best friend. (See Chapter 10 for more about carbs and sleep.)

Choosing the right carbs also can make your day. a twofold increase in serotonin levels means you are most likely to crawl out of the emotional dumpster and laugh off an insult. It means thinking more positively, so you appreciate a break in the clouds rather than focus on how cold it is. It means joy instead of doom and gloom. It means feeling as happy and energetic in the winter as you do with the sunshine of summer.

The More You Lose, the Better You Feel

Choosing the right carbs also is an important step in dropping unwanted pounds. For one thing, it means you won't be tempted to binge and can pass on the pretzels or other treats at work and the buttered popcorn at night. Fewer pig-outs means fewer calories, and as calories drop, so does body fat.

The extra bonus is that the more weight you lose, the bigger the mood boost you get from eating carbs!

That's because as you lose unwanted body fat, your body's insulin becomes more efficient at normalizing blood sugar and moving amino acids into the muscles and out of the blood. That leaves more tryptophan behind to enter the brain and convert to serotonin. And as you know by now, the bigger the serotonin boost, the better your mood and the lower your carb cravings. In short, the longer you work with your serotonin, the more weight you will lose, the better you will feel and the easier it will be to lose more weight!

The solution is easy. You don't need to be ruled by your inner grouch. All you need to do is eat quality carbs in the right amounts.

Bye-Bye White Food

All carbs will boost your mood, since every one of them—from white bread to brown rice—is made up of long strands of glucose. However, only the quality carbs in whole grains and colorful starchy vegetables like sweet potatoes will give you sustained energy and a mood high without the extra calories and a blood sugar roller-coaster ride. Only whole grains help you manage weight and lower the risk for heart disease, diabetes, hypertension and possibly cancer.

You already know that processed grains are a nutritional wasteland. They are drained of most mood-boosting vitamins and minerals, and have lost most of their brain-protecting antioxidants.

How Much More Is in Whole Grains?

When compared to processed wheat, whole wheat has a ton more of just about every nutrient studied.

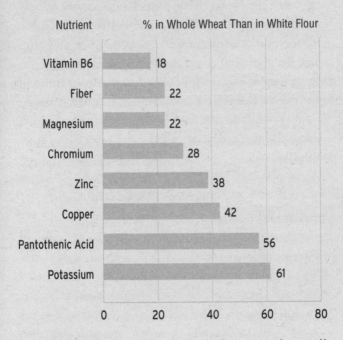

Nutrient	% in Whole Wheat Than in White Flour
Vitamin B6	18
Fiber	22
Magnesium	22
Chromium	28
Zinc	38
Copper	42
Pantothenic Acid	56
Potassium	61

In contrast, unprocessed whole grains have all three layers of the original grain—the nutrient-rich germ, the carb-packed endosperm and the fibery bran. No wonder whole grains are loaded with all their original nutrition, plus thousands of antioxidants, such as ferulic acid, caffeic acid, phytosterols, saponins, phenols and p-Coumaric acid, that protect the brain from damage and aging, and your mood from heading south. Phytates in whole grains deactivate cancer-causing substances. Phenols prevent cancer from attacking organs and tissues. Lignans are especially protective against breast cancer. Whole grains also are packed with nutrients that help the brain convert tryptophan into serotonin and that improve your chances of living a long and happy life. For example, one study found that the trace mineral chromium, found in whole grains, improved mood and lowered food cravings in depressed people. Hey, eating the right kind of bread (or cereal) could save your life!

Avoid the Blood Sugar Roller Coaster

It is not only just about what quality carbs do, but also what they *don't* do. Fiber-rich whole grains fill you up on fewer calories, so you *don't* stuff yourself to the point of being comatose. No wonder study after study has found that people who eat the most whole grains *don't* gain weight, *don't* develop diabetes and heart disease and *don't* need to worry as much about high blood pressure or even cancer. Combine whole grains with a calorie-controlled diet and studies show you boost brain power and lower inflammatory factors, so you *don't* suffer from everything from dementia to heart disease. Scarf down refined grains and you get just the opposite: weight gain, bad moods and higher risks for disease.

How come whole grains help with weight loss, but refined grains cause weight gain? Whole grains have fiber. Fiber fills us up, so we eat less. Also, most truly 100% whole grains are lower in fat and sugar, so they have fewer calories. In contrast, without the fiber, refined grains don't fill us up. We eat too much, then feel stuffed and sluggish. I've heard it over and over again. When people eat processed grains, they overdo it, yet they don't feel satisfied. "I love pasta and pizza. But I don't have a 'full sensor' with either one. I can keep eating and eating, which in the long run leaves me miserable.... I call it the food hangover! It's weird, but regardless of how overly full I feel, pasta leaves me craving ice cream, while pizza leaves me craving soda, especially root beer. Go figure!" says Danielle, a track coach and teacher in Salem, Oregon.

Blood Sugar Boogie: The Glycemic Index

One of the reasons fiber-packed whole grains are waist-reducers is their scores on the glycemic index (GI). This index ranks foods on a scale of 1 to 100 by how quickly they convert to glucose and raise blood sugar levels. For example, pure glucose scores a 100, while low-fat/sugar-free yogurt or peanuts score about 14. The lower the number, the gentler the rise in blood sugar and the more likely a food will help with weight loss, mood and memory, as well as lower your risk for a host of other ills, including heart disease and diabetes. A diet loaded with high glycemic foods does just the opposite.

A score of 55 is the cutoff point: foods below this line are low-glycemic foods. As GI scores go up from this point, a food is considered more and more a mood and health risk. One study found that the more high-glycemic foods women ate, the worse their PMS symptoms. Another study found that people think more clearly when their diets are based on low-glycemic foods. On the other hand, people who eat lots of high-GI foods, especially if those foods also are high in calories (think white hamburger buns, French fries, toaster pastries, crackers, yada yada yada), typically are hungry more often. They also eat up to 700 calories more each day than do happy, fit people who turn to whole grains and low-GI foods for their carb fix. In addition, the more whole grains and other low-GI foods people eat, the sharper their minds, thinking and memories. It is a no-brainer. Why would you eat another refined grain when the benefits are so amazing for quality carbs?!

Many factors influence how fast the body digests a carb-rich food, but in general, whole grains and high-fiber foods rank lower on the GI scale than refined grains and processed foods. *A rule of thumb is the less processed a food, the lower its GI score and the more likely it will improve mood and help you lose weight.* For example,

- Old-fashioned oats have a GI score of 49, but instant oatmeal scores a 66.
- Brown rice scores 50, but instant white rice scores 87.
- Whole-wheat kernels score 30, while Instant Cream of Wheat scores 74.
- Whole-wheat spaghetti scores 32, but enriched spaghetti scores up to 64.

Consequently, shortly after eating a buttermilk freezer waffle (GI of 76), a slice of white bread (GI of up to 70), some fruit leather (GI of 90) or a handful of crackers (GI of 70), your plummeting blood sugar leaves you shaky, groggy and hungry. Simply making the switch from a processed grain to a whole grain can make a world of difference in your mood. Lindsey, the public relations exec in Minneapolis, found this out firsthand: "I made the switch from those gooey muffins at the coffee shop to whole grains I brought from home after I noticed that if I overdo the processed carbs throughout the day, they leave me feeling tired and crabby, not to mention bloated."

She's not alone. People often complain that a mid-morning or midafternoon carb-fest leaves them unable to focus, in a mental fog and searching for the nearest vending machine. The result? They eat too much of all the wrong stuff and gain weight. It's no wonder that eating refined grains increases diabetes risk more than twofold! Corn flakes with a GI ranking of 84 or potatoes at 93 wreak such havoc with blood sugar levels that some experts recommend placing these foods at the top of the Food Guide Pyramid along with sugar and other junk foods.

The glycemic index is pretty complicated, since a food's score will change based on other foods at the meal. GI scores vary from person to person and even fluctuate enormously in the same person from day to day. You also need to compare a food's GI score with the amount of calories and carbs in the food, a factor called the "glycemic load." For example, a potato has a high glycemic score and it packs a bunch of carbs, while carrots and watermelon have high GI numbers, but few calories or carbs. Rather than obsess about the numbers, the simple guideline for eating in tune with your blood sugar and your serotonin levels is to choose lots of fiber-rich foods, switch from potatoes to sweet potatoes, cut out the processed carbs and select whole grains in their least processed form.

How to Tell a Good Carb from a Bad One

If you haven't gotten the message yet, let's get one thing absolutely straight—your body and brain need carbs. This is the brain's number one fuel of choice and the kindling fuel that helps burn body fat. Eat less than 130 grams of carbs a day and I promise you will notice problems concentrating, remembering, learning and being creative. Your mood also is likely to take a nosedive.

It happened to me in the days when I was a foolish dieter who jumped on the first Atkin's fad back in the 1980s. I had been on that ridiculous low-carb diet for about two days when my friend Abby and I played a game of tennis. By the end of the first set, I was so energy drained, I couldn't finish the game. I went straight home and slept for 14 hours. I got up from that carb-depleted nap and ate half a loaf of French bread. That was the shortest diet I have ever been on!

All respected nutrition experts, from the USDA's Dietary Guidelines to the American Heart Association, recommend most people get somewhere between 45% to 65% of their calories from carbs. That is 225 to 325 grams for someone on a 2,000 calorie diet. To put that into perspective:

- A slice of bread averages about 15 grams of carbs.
- A banana has 27 grams.
- Two carrots have 12 grams.
- A serving of Minty Rice, Orange and Pomegranate Bowl (see Recipes section) has 53 grams.
- A cup of whole-grain cereal with milk and a small piece of fruit contain about 60 grams of carbs.
- A serving of Mashed Roasted Sweet Potatoes with a Taste of Honey (see Recipes section) has almost 40 grams.

- A serving of Nutty Green Tea Rice (see Recipes section) has almost 39 grams.
- A small bean burrito supplies about 36 grams.
- A cup of pasta with marinara sauce adds another 45 grams.

Complement those meals with salad, bread, fruit and yogurt, and it is easy to see how quickly the carb grams add up.

Happy, fit people choose most of their carbs from the high-quality category. Yet this is not quite as easy as it sounds. If you are a typical American, you average less than one whole grain a day. Look around you—more than nine out of every ten people within sight don't get even three whole grains in a day. You probably think you are getting more than this, but it is only because most foods appear to have more whole grains than they really do. For example, which of the following would you guess is a true-blue whole grain?

- Rudi's Organic Bakery Multigrain Oat Bread
- Wheat Thins Fiber Selects 5-Grain
- Nutri-Grain Cereal Bars
- Private Selection Organic Multigrain Waffles with no preservatives
- Honey Wheatberry Bread Oroweat

The answer? None.

Food companies are tripping all over themselves trying to come up with ways to capitalize on the whole-grain trend, yet they still offer foods that look and taste like the junk so many Americans have grown accustomed to. Many of the grains on grocery shelves might sound healthy, but are really junk in disguise. Terms on a label that mean absolutely nothing include

7-grain	wheat	sprouted wheat
multigrain	stoneground	wheat
wheatberry	rye	with whole wheat
cracked wheat	oatmeal	

On labels, only "100%" is 100% reliable. Unless a bread or cereal says 100% whole grain, don't believe anything on the front of a label. Even white bread can call itself wheat bread, since the main ingredient is wheat flour, which is refined flour. Always turn the package over and look at the nutritional panel and ingredient list on the back. A whole grain—such as whole wheat, oats, barley, millet or wheat flakes— should be the first ingredient, and ideally the words *enriched, refined* or *wheat flour* (all names for white flour) should be nowhere in sight. When it comes to fiber, look for at least 5 grams per serving for cereals and 2 grams per slice of bread or serving of rice, pasta or other packaged grains. (Your ultimate daily goal is at least 30 grams of fiber from whole grains, vegetables, fruits, nuts and legumes.)

Watch out for prepared, packaged grains with exotic flavors—they can come at a high fat or sodium cost. A cup of Rice-a-Roni or Uncle Ben's Caribbean Black Beans and Rice tallies up to half your day's maximum sodium quota in one serving. One serving of Hormel's Compleats Chicken Alfredo has 1,300 milligrams and their Chicken and Noodles has 1,400 milligrams of sodium—that is your entire day's recommended allotment for salt!

Don't use blind faith even with your favorite brands—they can be deceiving. Some brands, such as Kashi, make some wonderful, high-fiber whole-grain cereals, but other products in the line, such as some of their crackers, have more white flour than whole and too much sodium.

Choose boxed whole grains that supply no more than 480 milligrams of sodium (which is still too high, but you'll be hard-pressed to find any lower than this). Products that meet this goal include

- Bellybar Mellow Oat snack bar
- Ancient Harvest Quinoa
- instant brown rice

Of course, even a bran muffin made with 100% organic whole wheat flour can still be an overly greasy, sweet treat, so use a bit of common sense when choosing whole grains. Always, always check the ingredient list and add up the numbers in the nutritional panel.

How Much Do You Really Need?

My guess is that if you are overweight or frequently feel a bit testy or grumpy, it is not just *what* you eat, but also *how* much.

In the past couple of decades, Americans have increased their daily calories by a whopping 15%, or about 300 more calories today than we ate back in the mid-1980s. We are eating 100 acres of pizza a day and 6.6 billion pounds of salty snacks like chips— 22 pounds a year for every man, woman and child. The average American now gobbles four orders of French fries a week.

Serving sizes for starch have expanded just as fast as Americans' waistlines. The average muffin is the size of a softball, not the recommended ping-pong ball. In a segment I did for ABC's *Good Morning America,* one take-out serving of spaghetti totaled 16 servings of grain, and that does not count the two slices of garlic bread that came with the order!

Basically, we are gorging on mountains of junk carbs, and as a result we feel worse and are getting fatter and fatter. It is no wonder that 70 million Americans don't sleep well, one in four battle the blues, almost 123 million are on serotonin-boosting medications and more than 6 out of every 10 of us are overweight!

One-Ounce Limit

While you need a few hundred grams of carbs a day to fuel your mind and body, it only takes 30 grams to get a serotonin boost. That is the equivalent of 1 to 1½ ounces of quality carbs. Even then, eat slowly. It takes about 20 to 30 minutes for the carb in your mouth to make it through the digestive tract and encourage tryptophan levels to rise in the brain. Have a light all-carb snack a half hour before you face off with the boss, give a nerve-racking presentation, go to bed or anticipate a carb craving, and by the time you walk through the door or hit the hay, you'll feel calmer, more relaxed, happier and more composed.

That's just what I told Colleen to do, and the results were amazing. She brought two to three 30-gram carb snacks, bundled into snack bags, with her to work. She called these snacks her "serotonin arsenal." By confronting stress well-armed with her quality-carb stash, she curbed cravings, calmed her nerves and stopped the daily trips to the pretzel store. She lost 22 pounds in just three months. More important, she kept the weight off. "And I wasn't even trying to lose weight!" she says, beaming.

Happy Carbs: Just a Dab Will Do Ya

To maximize the serotonin boost, have a snack 30 minutes before you need to relax, go to bed, or your crave-prone time of the day. Limit the snack to about 150 to 200 calories, and 30 grams (1 ounce) of carbs, which is:

- A whole-grain muffin the size of a ping-pong ball
- 4 cups of air-popped popcorn (lightly salt it to make a great alternative to potato chips)
- 2 slices of cinnamon raisin bread
- 100% whole wheat English muffin with 2 teaspoons jam
- 5 graham crackers
- 9 Triscuits
- 75 100% whole-grain thin pretzel sticks
- 1 thin slice of angel food cake topped with ¼ cup berries

10 Steps for a Carb Makeover

If you are a carb craver, you need to treat yourself with a little kindness. It's not your fault you can't keep your fingers out of the cookie jar or the bag of chips. You can't "will away" those cravings. They are hardwired in your head.

So work with your carb cravings. Make sure each meal contains at least one whole grain. Plan a quality-carb snack at your most craving-prone time of the day (typically midafternoon or late evening). To maximize your mood and minimize your weight, you need to take this quality-carb message seriously. That means tackling the issue with a 10-step plan.

Step #1. Purge the kitchen of all white flour. Open the cupboards and toss the junk. Throw out the obvious: the white rice, the instant mashed potatoes, any cracker or cookie made with anything but 100% whole grain (you are pretty much down to Triscuits and 100% Whole Wheat Fig Newtons), all potato chips, Pop-Tarts, boxes of bread crumbs, Pasta Roni, Hamburger Helper, cans of Chef Boyardi Ravioli, Costco muffins and such. Search the freezer for French fries, hash browns, breakfast foods made from processed grains or other high-calorie/low-quality items like Marie Callender's frozen pasta entrees or pot pies.

Definitely toss your carb triggers, junk foods that you are powerless to resist. Remember, if you have to drive to the store to get ice cream, you will be much less likely to binge.

Then read labels on the rest. If wheat flour or enriched flour is in the top three ingredients on a label, you are holding a poor-quality carb. Toss it.

Okay, okay, if this cold-turkey approach is a bit over the top, then keep two or three junk carbs and toss the rest. But beware: these items may be "trigger" foods that tempt you to indulge. Also, keep in mind that *this is not so much about "giving up" as it is "giving to" your health, your mood, and your belly and thighs.*

Step #2. Restock the kitchen with the 100% whole grains you like, such as 100% whole-wheat bread, old-fashioned oatmeal, Kashi Autumn Wheat Cereal or GoLean Cereal, Zoom hot cereal or instant brown rice. Experiment with new grains, like barley, millet, amaranth, whole-wheat couscous or bulgur.

If you can't imagine your spouse or kids loving whole-wheat pasta or whole-wheat tortillas, then choose the next best thing. For example, try Aunt Jemima frozen Pancakes with Whole Grains, or tortillas or pastas made from blends of whole wheat and refined wheat, such as Ronzoni or Barilla whole-wheat blend pastas.

Step #3. Switch to quality carbs in recipes. For example, if a recipe calls for

white rice: use instant brown or wild rice, bulgur, millet or other whole grains

flour: use at least half whole-wheat flour

bread (such as French toast): use whole-grain bread

potatoes: use sweet potatoes, yams, squash and/ or corn

Step #4. Plan snacks and bring grains with you. When packing your lunch and snacks for the day, make sandwiches with 100% whole-grain bread, use low-fat cheeses such as Cabot Vermont 50% Reduced

Fat Cheese, and include other grains like 100% whole-grain crackers or air-popped popcorn.

Step #5. Create nonfood rewards. Praise yourself with a manicure, flowers, a game of golf on Saturday or a Netflix movie. Follow the "if…then" rule: *if* you steer clear of the junk, *then* you get the back rub, hour of alone time or bubble bath.

Step #6. Take time. Often we grab food before we even know whether we really want it. That knee-jerk reaction gets us into trouble. Take a 10-minute pause before diving into any snack, from popcorn to leftover doughnuts.

Step #7. Identify the craving. Is it for something crunchy or chewy? Cold, sweet or creamy? Once you have pinpointed exactly what you want, then find a low-calorie food that satisfies that craving. Luckily, the better you eat, the more your cravings for fatty or overly sweet carbs will dwindle.

Step #8. Eat breakfast. As discussed in Chapter 2, eat a nutritious breakfast and you are much more likely to resist junk-food temptations throughout the day.

Step #9. Keep hunger at bay. Eat small meals and snacks evenly distributed throughout the day. This helps keep serotonin levels (and other nerve chemicals like NPY) in the normal range.

Step #10. Out of sight, out of mind. Put another way, seeing is craving. Watch out for temptations at the mall, restaurants and friends' houses. It is easy to overdo carbs when most of the ones offered to you are the low-quality ones. For example, studies at the University of Illinois found that people ate 45% more calories when there was a bread basket placed on the table in restaurants than when the waiter came by and offered them a slice from a basket. Ask that the tortilla chips be removed when dining at a Mexican restaurant and you will save yourself 300 unnecessary calories. Avoid the coffee shop with the display of muffins, scones and croissants.

Habit, Not Chemistry

Not all cravings are caused by serotonin. Sometimes we eat out of habit. If potato chips midafternoon taste good, you are likely to have it again. Repeating the snack over and over, day after day, results in a habit or even a craving.

In these cases, take charge by substituting a more nutritious snack. Replace the midmorning doughnut with a small whole-wheat bagel, exchange the afternoon chips with air-popped popcorn, or swap out the evening ice cream for low-fat custard-style yogurt or frozen blueberries. Or you can develop a new habit to replace the old one, such as taking a walk during your high-craving time of the day or riding an exercise bicycle instead of snacking while watching television.

Think big. You want to feel good today and great in the future. The longer you take good care of yourself, working with your body and its natural rhythms, the better you will feel, the more energy you will have and the sharper your mind and memory will be. The more improvements you make in your diet, the faster and the more amazing the results. But any change, no matter how small, if you stick with it, will help boost mood, thinking and energy. That's what happy, fit people have learned to do, one step at a time.

Be patient. You can't expect pasta to work like Prozac, at least not immediately. It will take two to three weeks of eating well before you will notice an improvement in your mood and cravings. Each day is one step. Make sure it is in the right direction.

SECRET 4:
ADOPT THE 6% SOLUTION

The Promise

**In one week of making
this change, you will:**

- notice a change
  in sugar cravings
- begin to appreciate
  the flavor of foods

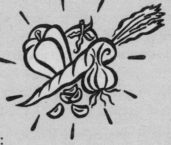

In one month, you will:

- experience more energy and a more steady energy level
  throughout the day
- feel less stressed
- be free from sweet cravings
- drop a few pounds
- notice an improvement in mood
- focus your attention and think more clearly

In one year, you will:

- lose up to 50 pounds
- have lowered your risk for many degenerative diseases,
  including heart disease, diabetes and high blood pressure

When Keli was a kid, one way her mom showed her how much she was loved was to give her cola at every meal, something her parents had been too poor to afford when Keli's mom was young. By the time Keli was in grade school, sugar was a diet staple. Cinnamon rolls crammed her eyes open in the morning, candy bars fueled her day, and cookies and more cola were her treats at night. In college, she needed those sugary treats just to calm her nerves, focus her attention to study and boost her lagging energy levels: "In those days, I was convinced that if it hadn't been for sugar, my high-strung personality would never have been able to cope with life."

Teasing about her diet, a friend challenged Keli to give up sugar for a month. Every time she caved to the sugar temptation by grabbing a doughnut or a candy bar, she'd have to start all over, beginning at day one. "It was horrible at first," she says. "My nerves were on edge. I was cranky and desperate for a sugar fix." Several times she made it a few days, gave into the craving for sugar and had to begin again. But, she says, "I'm a pretty competitive person, so I was determined to prove that I could do it."

And she did. By the end of the sugar-free month, Keli was a new woman. That nervous personality melted away. The inability to focus and the energy highs and lows she always had experienced and thought were just her lot in life were really just riding the swells of runaway blood sugar. She now says, "I never knew who I really was because I'd always been either on a sugar high or a sugar crash. Once I'd cut all sugar out of my diet, I found I really liked myself. I was energetic but not frantic. I was calm, collected, smart and even sometimes downright wise."

Drowning in Sweet

Like Keli, most of us haven't a clue how much sugar we eat or how it affects our moods, energy level, weight and lives. The U.S. Department of Agriculture (USDA) reports we drench ourselves in 30 to 50 teaspoons of added sugar every day (and that's not counting the natural sugars in milk, fruit or other unprocessed foods). "Sugar intake rose rapidly from the 1960s to 1999, when it dropped a bit. But Americans still average about 142 pounds per person every year," says Steve Haley, the sugar expert at the USDA.

Think about it—we swallow approximately 30 teaspoons of sugar per day. That's 497 calories a day (the calorie equivalent of a hamburger and fries!), more than 25% of a person's dietary intake from a substance that provides *nothing* but calories and heartache. Put another way, if all you gave up dietwise was added sugars, you'd lose 50 pounds in a year!

We Are Born to Love Sugar

Our affair with sugar begins with a kiss. The tongue has up to 10,000 tastebuds, each one programmed to detect the taste of either sweet, sour, bitter or salty. Yet it is the tastebuds wired for sugar that hold the most prestigious spot—right up front on the tip of the tongue. We inherited this sweet tooth from our most ancient ancestors as one of our many survival skills—sweet foods are typically safe foods that also pack a nice calorie load, while bitter foods are more often toxic or poisonous. The smart cave dwellers who figured that out lived to reproduce. We are their offspring.

Our brains evolved chemicals to further entice us to relish sweets. Studies at Johns Hopkins University and elsewhere have found that the very taste of sugar on the tongue releases morphinelike chemicals in the brain, called endorphins, that calm jittery nerves and produce a natural high. (By the way, you also get an endorphin rush from meditation, laughing really hard or exercise.) It is the taste of sweet that calms babies, entices kids to eat Count Chocula cereal and warms the hearts of lovers. For the love of sweet, prehistoric hunter-gatherers drew pictures of figs and dates on cave walls, Egyptians kept bees as far back as 2,600 B.C. and the Promised Land was said to flow with milk and honey. We have been head over heels in love with sugar for a long, long time.

All of us are programmed to love sugar. Nothing could be more natural and more normal. According to a study from Tufts University, almost all of us crave a sweet treat at least once in a while, regardless of whether we are fat or thin, happy or sad, young or old, relaxed or stressed. Sugar, in the tiny amounts nibbled by our ancestors, even makes us happy! But, like folks who are hardwired for alcoholism, abuse that natural sugar high and you are headed for trouble with a capital T.

The Natural High

Our bodies are designed to love sweets. Work with that natural instinct by including small amounts of quality sweets in your weekly diet and you'll improve your mood without sacrificing your waistline.

Is Sugar Addictive?

With all that wiring for sweet, including brain chemicals that entice us to eat it and tastebuds that tell us it is delicious, it's no surprise that some people say they are addicted to the stuff. Sugar is our number one comfort food, which explains why cranky premenstrual women turn to sugar with a vengeance, increasing their daily intake by as much as 20 teaspoons a day (for a total of 50 teaspoons!). Alcoholics in recovery reach for sweets and caffeine to counter their depression, fatigue and irritability. People trying to quit cigarettes do the same.

For years, experts said there was no such thing as a sugar addict; our love of sugar was merely habit, not addiction. Research from Princeton University changed all that. These studies showed that animals fed high-sugar diets exhibited all the symptoms of withdrawal, including agitation and nervousness, when sugar was taken away. Autopsies also showed brain changes that mimicked drug addiction. "Reintroduce sugar to their diets and the animals binge, all of which are classic symptoms of substance abuse," says Bartley Hoebel, Ph.D., Professor of Psychology at Princeton and lead researcher on the studies.

The researchers also found that even after sugar is removed from the diet, it takes at least two weeks before withdrawal symptoms subside. Dr. Hoebel adds that sugar is by no means as powerful a drug as heroin. He prefers to call it a dependency, rather than an addiction. Other researchers disagree, citing studies on animals that show sugar is more addicting than cocaine.

One reason why sugar is so habit-forming is that it turns on our bodies' own heroin-like chemicals, the endorphins. The very taste of sugar on the tongue releases endorphins in the brain, and these cousins to heroin or morphine are highly addictive. The body likes this high and wants to repeat it, so the brain releases another nerve chemical called dopamine that permanently stamps the experience into our memory banks to entice us to seek this yummy taste again. The response is so powerful that even the sight of the food, let alone the smell, at a later date will release dopamine and a craving for another taste and mood fix.

Sugar also has a calming, comforting effect when we are stressed, which only adds to its addictive potential. Mary Dallman, Ph.D. at the University of California, San Francisco, found that animals who feasted on sugar when stressed showed a lower stress response compared to rats fed regular chow. "What was fascinating about these findings was that without sugar, the rats' stress response stayed high," says Dr. Dallman. The rats needed the sugar to calm down; without it, they remained stressed out.

The stress hormones, cortisol in particular, apparently prompt the typical fight-or-flight response to anything threatening, but also scramble appetite-control chemicals like serotonin, NPY and the endorphins that signal the brain to seek calorie-packed foods. These foods, in turn, calm us down and rein in the stress. In essence, we are turning to foods to self-medicate.

That's what happened to Taryn, a housewife in Oregon. Her cravings for sweetened oatmeal escalated into a binge during the years her marriage was spiraling downhill. The more stressed she got, the more bowls of sweet carbs she ate, until the binges sometimes monopolized entire days. Then the panic attacks began. "Within days of separating from my husband and not living with those constant judgmental attacks, the uncontrollable cravings began to subside," she says. She hasn't had a panic attack and has been binge-free for 10 years.

Those cookie-loving rats, however, also gain weight and really pack on belly fat, probably because cortisol is very bossy about where the body should store fat during stress. The same has been shown in other studies on humans: we eat more sweets when anxious, with ice cream being the number one favorite comfort food. As a result, we gain more weight, especially around the middle. That belly fat is a highway to heart disease, diabetes, high blood pressure, possibly cancer and the metabolic syndrome. While sweet comfort foods apply the brakes on chronic stress, helping us cope and feel better when times are rough, in the long run they make us miserable and fat.

Don't Be Duped!

The food industry uses that natural-born, hardwired, genetically programmed desire for sugar to turn a diet once sprinkled with a bit of sweet into a wasteland of oversweetened junk.

For all of human history, dating back hundreds of thousands of years, sugar has been a minor player in the diet. Originally, people chewed sugarcane, then sometime around 350 A.D., folks in India invented a way to extract sugar from plants. Even then, sugar remained an infrequent treat, not a daily occurrence. As recently as the early 1900s, sugar was bought directly by the consumer for homemade jams and the occasional pie. That means people like my grandmother living in Banks, Oregon, in 1910 sprinkled about 4 teaspoons of sugar into each of her sons' daily meals, for a total of 64 calories coming from added sugar or about 13 pounds of sweet a year.

Fast-forward to the present, where 3 out of every 4 teaspoons is added to processed foods before they reach our kitchens, and every man, woman and child averages somewhere between 100 and 142 pounds a year, or 2 to 3 pounds of added sugar a week! That's between 181,600 and 257,872 empty calories every year. If you are having a hard time wrapping your mind around that number, try this: Line up 20 5-pound bags of pure sugar on your kitchen counter. Stand back and take a good, long look at how much added sugar each person in your family is likely to eat from one birthday to the next. It's astounding!

You Eat More Than You Think

My guess is you eat a lot more added sugar than you think. It's obvious that Frosted Flakes, soft drinks and jelly beans have sugar. It's easy to taste the sugar in a cookie, a tablespoon of jam or a squirt of pancake syrup. But a whole bunch of sugar in American diets comes from processed foods that aren't even sweet, from canned chili, frozen turkey entrees, pizza, peanut butter and bread to hot dogs, baked beans, canned soups and salad dressings. For example,

- half a cup of canned creamed-style corn has almost 2 teaspoons of added sugar.
- Weight Watchers Smart Ones Teriyaki Chicken and Vegetables or a serving of canned beans and franks has more than 3 teaspoons.
- A Hot Pockets Cheeseburger has 3.5 teaspoons.
- A cup of canned ravioli or an Odwalla bar both have 4 teaspoons.
- Marie Callender's Fettucine Alfredo with Garlic Bread has almost 5 teaspoons.

I did a segment for ABC's *Good Morning America* that addressed the question, "How harmful is all the candy kids eat at Halloween?" The take-home message was that if we limited the candy binge to just Halloween and Easter, there would be no problem with the amount of sugar we are eating. But kids and adults are eating the sugar equivalent of a huge bag of candy every day, 365 days of the year, year after year after year. The example I gave on the show was a typical, reasonably nutritious-appearing menu that included

For breakfast: a packet of flavored oatmeal, canned fruit and milk

For lunch: beans and franks, sweetened applesauce, chocolate milk and two small cookies

For dinner: spaghetti, salad with dressing, cranberry juice and frozen yogurt

The day's food intake totaled 46.8 teaspoons (187.2 grams) of added sugar—the equivalent of 17 mini Musketeers bars!

Carb, Schmarb: Who Cares If It's Sugar or Starch?

Sugar is just a carbohydrate and, as we talked about in Chapter 3, carbs boost serotonin levels and that makes us relaxed and happy. So what's the big deal?

The problem is that while sugar is a carbohydrate, it is a poor substitute for the carbs in whole-wheat bread or brown rice. Think of it as a big bowl of grease. Sure, it will supply calories and keep you alive, but you won't live well or long.

Carbs are divided into two camps: complex and simple. Complex carbs in oatmeal or sweet potatoes are long strings of sugar connected together like a string of pearls or a line of boxcars on a train. Your body can't use them this way, so they must be digested, or broken down into their individual sugar units (pearls or cars) before they are absorbed and used for fuel in the body. That breakdown process happens in the gut and takes time, so quality carbs enter the bloodstream slowly, causing a gentle rise in blood sugar. As a result, your body has the energy it needs to think, jog or keep your heart beating. You stay full and satisfied and are less likely to overeat later in the day. As mentioned in Chapter 3, people who eat the most quality carbs are the ones who are most likely to stay slim. And what happy, fit people have learned is that when they switch from sugar to whole grains, they work with their bodies' natural balance. They cut calories and lose weight, while boosting their energy and mood. What a deal!

In contrast, simple carbs or sugars are ready for immediate use, so they require no digestion and are absorbed quickly, raising blood sugar levels too high, too fast. They are high–glycemic index (GI) foods.

Most high-sugar foods jack up blood sugar levels faster than you can say "more sugar, please." High blood sugar levels trigger the release of the hormone insulin, which shuttles the sugar out of the blood. But, like any high-GI food, when blood sugar levels are too high, insulin often overreacts, removing too much sugar from the blood and converting that sugar into fat for storage, rather than using it for energy. Low blood sugar, in turn, leaves you jittery, hungry and irritable. You eat again and the cycle continues, leading to a roller-coaster ride of blood sugar highs and lows and the addition of lots of jiggly fat on your hips, thighs and belly.

This explains why studies show we eat up to 53% more calories after a high-GI snack compared to a quality carb snack with a low-GI score. Victoria, a health writer in Beaverton, Oregon, knows this firsthand:

"My husband and I got a bit out of control with sugar a few years back. We noticed that the more often we gave in to temptation, the more often we craved sugar. We gave up sugar cold-turkey, well, except for our Saturday night dessert. The first two weeks were really hard. I craved sugar desperately and even had headaches, which I attributed to my sugar 'detox.' It got a lot easier after that and I felt so much better...and I dropped 11 pounds over the next two months."

What's Low Blood Sugar Feel Like?

Eat a sugary snack, then watch your body react. If you experience any of the following symptoms within an hour, your blood sugar probably has dropped.

Apathy	Depression	Disorientation
Fatigue	Forgetfulness	Headache
Shakiness	Irritability	Lightheadedness
Moody feelings	Poor memory	Poor judgment

Sugar Makes You Fat

You've probably heard that all carbohydrates—whether they come from a candy bar, brown rice or an apple—have 4 calories per gram. That's only true in theory. Pure carbs from any source are all the same caloriewise. In the real world, however, carbs are diluted in whole grains, fruits or starchy vegetables because of the water and fiber. Processed sugary foods don't have that fiber and water—they are just concentrated calories. Ounce for ounce, pure sugar has about four times more calories than an ounce of cooked rice or an apple slice. In case that didn't completely sink in, let me repeat that: processed sweets supply four times more calories compared to real fruit because the sugar molecules are diluted by all the juice and crunch in the real food.

To make matters worse, most added sugars are typically found in foods that are also dripping with fat, such as cookies, muffins, cakes, ice cream, candy bars, granola bars, and the like. Study after study shows that the more sugar animals and people eat, the greater the likelihood they will be fat. In turn, the heavier we are, the more sugar we want. Even when the calories are identical, a person who gets more of those calories from sugar will pack on the pounds faster than you can say "Snickers Bar." One study from the University of Southern California found that the more sugar a person ate, the greater the risk for obesity and insulin insensitivity, a risk factor for diabetes. Another study from the University of Alabama found that even limiting sugar to 10% of calories isn't enough to prevent weight gain or diabetes, heart disease and memory loss.

On the other hand, happy, fit people have learned it is easier to lose weight when they cut back on sugar. For example, Alex, the college student in Washington, says, "I've lost 60 pounds and have kept the weight off since I've been in college. I know that cutting out sugar was a huge reason for my success. I can't have just one bite of a cookie. If I do, I eat the whole bag, so saying no to the temptation in the first place makes keeping the weight off so much easier for me."

Don't get me wrong. Sugar by itself doesn't cause weight gain or a bad mood. Besides, it's only natural to feel out of sorts at times and turn to ice cream or a doughnut to soothe a blue mood, say, for example, when you can't fit into last year's swimsuit or when you argue with a loved one. Feeling funky is all part of the ups and downs of life. Reaching for a bit of sugar to help when you are tearing your hair out can be soothing and certainly won't hurt. Most happy, fit people satisfy their sweet tooths now and then. In fact, we are designed to indulge in a bit of sugar on occasion. Sweets are one of life's best natural highs. The problem is not what, but how much and how often. It is the glut of sugar that is bringing us down—mood- and weightwise.

Sugar is a Downer

Don't you just love those commercials where thin, vibrant, beautiful young people are frolicking on the beach? They stop briefly from their bouncy game of volleyball or after surfing the ultimate wave to grab a candy bar for a quick energy boost. The ad ends with the question, "Why take time out of your busy life when all you need is a Booster Bar to keep your life on track?" What a bunch of hooey! The last thing you need to boost your energy level is a sugar-drenched, highly processed wad of junk food!

As Keli found out when she went cold-turkey on sugar, foods packed with this highly processed sweetener send you down the road to grumpville. Oh sure, sugar can boost serotonin levels in much the same way as quality carbs. But unlike their high-fiber counterparts, sweet treats are a short-term fix. In the long run, they are downers. Within 30 minutes of the sugar rush, your blood sugar plummets and you crash faster than a plane out of gas. The grog period lingers, leaving you drowsy for several hours afterwards.

While quality grains are a big help in beating depression, sugar actually aggravates the funk. Studies from the University of South Alabama found that, unlike those perky, sugar-gorging beach lovers, many people battling fatigue and depression report improvements in energy levels within a week or two of eliminating sugar from their diets. As the fatigue lifts, so does depression. The researchers concluded that compared to the temporary high people get from sugar, eliminating sugar from the diet is a permanent solution to depression for many people.

You might be thinking, "Hey, this isn't my problem. I'm healthy and fit, so why should I care about this sugar thing?" You need to care because even though these studies were on people with clinical depression, the researchers say that anyone who is sensitive to sugar would benefit since they probably would experience the grumps somewhere down the road as a result of their sugar intakes.

We all know some happy, skinny chick who lives on doughnuts, or some muscle-bound dude on an all-cookie diet. Those people are exceptions, not the rule. Those four or five people in the whole world who seem oblivious to sugar are freaks. For the vast majority of us, our health and waistlines are buckling under the weight of sugar in our diets. Besides, even if you are one of the few people who is at their ideal body weight, too much sugar still could increase your risk for blood sugar problems, fatigue and possibly even weight gain down the road. Everyone, lean or fat, happy or sad, should heed the sugar wake-up call when it comes to health.

From Cavities to Cancer

Everyone knows that a high-sugar diet causes all kinds of dental problems. But this is just the tip of the iceberg. A study from the University of British Columbia found that high-sugar diets turn off a gene that regulates levels of sex hormones, like testosterone and estrogen, increasing a person's risk for a host of ills, from acne and infertility to polycystic ovaries and uterine cancer. According to the American Heart Association, overly sweet diets raise blood triglyceride levels while lowering HDLs, the good cholesterol, thus increasing heart-disease risk. Other studies found that excessive sugar intake increases risk for pancreatic cancer, breast cancer and diabetes. Many researchers also suspect a sugar-laden diet is a culprit in the development and progression of depression and mood swings, memory loss, fatigue, osteoporosis, vision loss and kidney disease. It's even been linked to pregnancy complications and birth defects.

Every time you shove some highly processed food packed with sugar in your mouth, you miss the opportunity to nourish your body with super mood foods loaded with brain-boosting nutrients, such as colorful vegetables, fresh fruit, whole grains, legumes, nuts and soy or low-fat dairy products. The more sugar you eat, the greater your chances of being malnourished.

The 6% Solution

What do a tall Mocha Frappuccino at Starbucks, a packet of pancake syrup at McDonald's, an 8-ounce tub of fruited yogurt, or a half cup of Ben & Jerry's Chocolate Fudge Brownie have in common? They all meet or exceed your daily added sugar quota for the entire day. In fact, order a bran muffin and a grande Mocha Frappuccino and your added sugar totals almost 18 teaspoons, or more than twice most people's entire day's quota.

One out of every four calories (25%) in most American diets comes from sugar. The World Health Organization recommends no more than 10%, and preferably 6%, of calories should come from added sugars. Studies show that when even 9% of calories come from added sugar, it is a red flag for weight and health problems. So, the lower limit of 6% is the best target. For a 2,000 calorie diet, that equates to 30 grams or 7½ teaspoons a day.

The more sensitive you are to sugar, the more important it is to give it up and the greater the benefits will be when you do. The more added sugar you eliminate from your diet and the faster you make the changes, the more dramatic will be the results in weight loss, improvements in mood and increased energy. The good news is, the longer you steer clear of sugar, the less tempted you will be to go back. You will feel so much better and, like any drug, your cravings will fade with time. "Once I got over the initial hump, avoiding sugar got easier and easier. I feel so great now, there is no way I will ever go back to being a sugar addict," says Keli.

Real versus Added Sugar

Let's get one thing perfectly clear right now. We are talking *added* sugar, not *natural* sugar. You only need to focus on added sugar. Naturally occurring sugars in real foods, like fructose in fresh fruit or lactose in plain milk or yogurt, is not an issue. The tiny amount of sugar in an apple or a glass of milk comes packaged with a ton of nutrients. These sugars typically have low-glycemic index scores, producing a slow and moderate rise in blood sugar. An apple is loaded with fiber and is so packed with phytonutrients that it has the antioxidant equivalent of 1,000 milligrams of vitamin C. Milk is a great source of protein, calcium and vitamin D, and also has zinc, magnesium, B vitamins and more. Both have diluted calories because of their high water content. For example, compare a carrot with a candy bar. The carrot has 30 calories, tons of beta-carotene, fiber, water and potassium, while the candy bar is just a 250-calorie land mine of sugar and fat.

It is *added* sugars that cause weight gain and disease. It is the *added* sugars that turn you into a tired, crabby grump. It is the *added* sugars that we can't control, often eating anything sweet that isn't nailed down. It is the *added* sugars that happy, fit people have set a limit on. And, unless you are a diabetic, it is only *added* sugars that should be counted gram by gram. In short, added sugars bring you down, while naturally sweet foods like grapes, oranges and mangoes help you lose weight and stay happy. If Mother Nature put sugar in a food, then it is good. If people put it there, then it's not so good.

Food manufacturers have used this added-versus-natural issue to their advantage, trying to convince you their sugary junk is made with real ingredients. For example, products sweetened with high-fructose corn syrup are touted as "natural" sugar, when in fact this overly sweet sugar has contributed to America's growing obesity epidemic.

Sugar Stats

- **30 teaspoons:** the average intake of added sugar daily for every man, woman and child in the United States
- **11 teaspoons:** the maximum added sugar allotment advised by the World Health Organization
- **16:** the number of calories in a teaspoon of sugar
- **4:** the number of grams in a teaspoon
- **10 to 11 teaspoons:** the amount of added sugar in a 12-ounce can of soda

Navigating the Sugar War Zone

How can you tell a natural sugar from an added one? You can't. At least not from the nutrition panel on a food label, since companies are required to only provide the total sugar content, not where the sugar came from. You must be a sleuth and go to the next best thing—the ingredient list. Even then, sugar comes disguised under a slew of aliases, including:

brown sugar	malt syrup
fructose	sugar
invert sugar	crystalline frustose
rice syrup	high-fructose corn syrup
corn sweetener	molasses
fruit juice concentrates	syrup
maltose	dextrose
sucrose	honey
corn syrup	raw sugar
glucose	

By law, a food's contents must be listed on the label in descending order from most to least. The nearer to the top of the list, the more of an ingredient is in the food. Manufacturers know you are smart and might check this out. They know sugar will be at the top of the list if they add a big dump of one type of sugar into their foods—and that you are smart enough to figure that out. So they take advantage of a label loophole: they add different sugars in smaller amounts, which sinks each sugar a little lower on the list, even though the total added sugar content is still massively high. Even a savvy shopper has no way to tally the total amount of sugars when they are buried throughout the ingredient list. For example, a ready-to-eat cereal might have no sugar in the top three ingredients, but farther down the list are sugar, brown sugar, corn syrup solids, honey and maltose. Tricky, huh?

What can you do? The rule of thumb when reading labels on any processed food that comes in a carton, bag, box, pouch or bottle is to skip any food

1. that contains sugar (or any of its aliases) in the top three ingredients, or
2. with several mentions of sugar throughout the list

On the other hand, don't...

- be fooled by new reduced-sugar foods, such as Frosted Flakes, which have just as many calories and carbs as their full-sugar counterparts (the sugar has been replaced with more refined flour!).
- worry about natural sugars in fruit, vegetables, plain yogurt or milk, since these sugars come packaged with vitamins, minerals, phytonutrients, fiber and/or protein.
- switch to "natural" sugars, such as honey, brown sugar, raw sugar, rice or agave syrups or turbinado. The dusting of nutrients in these sugars makes nary a dent in your dietary needs. (It takes 15 cups of honey—containing

15,450 calories—to supply the calcium in one cup—90 calories—of nonfat milk.)

- be fooled by healthy-sounding foods, like fruited yogurt, bottled fruit smoothies, granola bars or super-fruit drinks or by the words *natural* or *organic* on the label.

- fall victim to foods labeled as "made with real fruit." You might see a strawberry or banana on the label, but none in the bag. Whether it's a breakfast bar or a candy bar, most of these products have little or none of the nutrition, fiber and phytonutrients of real fruit. Manufacturers put a drop of juice into the product, then flavor it with sugar, oil and colorings, yet call it fruit. Same goes for products that say on the label they are "made with real fruit juice." In most cases, added sugar outweighs fruit.

What about all those "natural" sweeteners? Count them as part of your added sugar quota. Teaspoon for teaspoon, barley malt and brown rice syrup have more calories than refined white sugar. Turbinado is less processed, but it still is added sugar, while molasses is slightly more nutritious, but these days it is made from a mix of molasses and refined sugar. Lo Han comes from a Chinese fruit but has a bitter, metallic aftertaste and has not been approved by the FDA. Agave nectar or syrup is an extract from a Mexican plant. It is mostly fructose and is sweeter than honey, so you can use less and it might have a lower glycemic index than other sugars. But it also has little research to prove it any safer or more nutritious than other sweeteners.

The Low-Down on Sugar Substitutes

No-cal sweeteners let you have your cake and eat it, too, so to speak. From NutraSweet and saccharine to Splenda and Nutrinova, they supply the sweet without the calories. But are they really all they are cracked up to be? Your guess is as good as mine.

• **The Cons.** A study from Purdue University found that even though these sweeteners don't have calories, they cause weight gain in animals. The researchers speculate that the intense sweetness tricks the brain, telling it that calories are on their way when they aren't. The body is confused, slows metabolism and amps up appetite. The end result is an imbalance in regulating calories that leads to overeating. In addition, not all have been cleared for safety. For example, stevia (including Only Sweet, a stevia product) is an extract from a South American shrub that has yet to be approved by the U.S. Food and Drug Administration as safe (studies show it might increase problems with the heart, kidneys and infertility). Others, such as Sweet Simplicity or Zsweet, might cause diarrhea.

• **The Pros.** A 2007 review of the research conducted by 10 universities and medical schools of more than 500 studies on aspartame, one of the leading no-cal sweeteners, found that it is safe even in high users and does not cause weight gain, cancer or nerve damage. Splenda has been studied for more than 20 years, has more than 100 studies to support its safety, and is approved for use in 80 countries. It is even safe for use by pregnant and nursing women.

> • **The Bottom Line.** Whether no-cal sweeteners help or hinder weight, one thing is certain: we are fatter today than we were 20 years ago despite the use of these sweeteners. Maybe for no other reason than people eat more food when they use these substitutes, with the attitude that "hey, I sweetened my coffee with Splenda, which means I can have a muffin!" For someone who must manage carb intake for health reasons, artificial sweeteners are a good idea. For everyone else, it's a good idea to use them in moderation.

17 Tips for the 6% Solution

Sugar is one of life's many pleasures. You can be happy and lean and also enjoy a little sugar in your diet. There is no need to give it up. Besides, the one time sugar is okay is when it encourages you to eat a super mood food (see Chapter 5 for details on the best mood-boosting, waist-slimming superfoods). You may need to cut back on, but not necessarily cut out, sugar. For some people, including anyone who is battling a weight problem, a mood issue, an energy drain or just eats too many sugary processed foods, that means wa-a-a-ay back.

The more sensitive your moods and cravings are to sugar, the bigger bang for your buck you'll get by cutting back. Highly processed, sugary items are the ultimate "dead" food. You deserve better than that. You deserve to be nourished and cared for. To feel vibrant and healthy. You won't get there eating a truckload of junk. You can become one of those happy, fit people if you make a few simple changes in your diet, one being to cut back on foods packed with added sugar.

Start by picking two of the following 17 tips. Practice those tips until they are habit, then return to the list to choose two more tips. Your goal is to adopt at least half or more of the following tips to break your sugar habit.

- **Tip #1: Focus on foods that are the biggest offenders.** More than 75% of America's sugar comes from soda and fruit drinks (we'll talk about them in Chapter 8), candy, sweet baked goods like cookies and muffins and ice cream. Most Americans would eliminate up to 78,000 calories and drop up to 20 pounds in a year by cutting these out of their diet.
- **Tip #2: Purge the kitchen of sugar.** Read labels on all boxed and bagged items in the cupboards, on the shelves and in the freezer and fridge. Throw out anything that fits those two basic rules: 1. sugar in the first three ingredients or 2. multiple sugars in the ingredient list. While you're at it, purge the dresser drawer, the closet and any other hiding places where you stash sugar. What's not in the house won't be eaten.
- **Tip #3: Desweeten recipes.** When baking, cut the amount of sugar by one-quarter or one-third. You won't even notice the difference

- **Tip #4: Control temptation.** Don't bring trigger foods into the house. If you are forced to have sugary foods at home, divvy them into individual serving-size baggies and place them out of sight.

- **Tip #5: Don't get over-hungry.** Eat breakfast, then eat regularly throughout the day. Bring healthy snacks with you, like air-popped popcorn or a few graham crackers, to nip temptation in the bud. People who divide their food intake into little meals and snacks work with their appetite centers, which helps them avoid fatigue, mood swings and uncontrollable cravings. It's no surprise nibblers are less prone to sugar cravings and have an easier time managing their weights.

- **Tip #6: Stick to the good stuff.** Why waste your sugar allowance on foods that aren't even sweet, like canned chili or a frozen entree? Skip the junk and focus on small amounts of the best desserts, which are most satisfying.

- **Tip #7: Stretch out the sweet treat to savor the experience.** Eat slowly. Focus on the flavor and experience of eating that thin slice of chocolate cake. Stop, put your fork down, and drink water in between bites. Choose sweets that take a long time to eat, such as a huge bowl of fresh strawberries dunked in a small dollop of chocolate syrup.

- **Tip #8: Split desserts.** Drink a cup of coffee instead of having a dessert or share a dessert with two other people.

- **Tip #9: Frantic for a sugar fix?** Then focus on the first one to three bites. This is where the endorphin rush kicks in and the tastebuds are soothed. After that, you're just pigging out.

- **Tip #10: Set ground rules.** Honor the old saying: fail to plan and you plan to fail! Establish rules about when and how you will indulge, such as not eating at the kitchen counter, out of the pie pan, off someone else's dessert plate or while watching TV. One ground rule is a must: never eat sugar on an empty stomach. The sugar shock will send you on a blood sugar roller-coaster ride that will wreak havoc with your mood and weight.

- **Tip #11: Boost serotonin levels with quality carbs.** You'll get the same serotonin boost with high-quality attitude adjusters, like whole grains, without the blood sugar drop. If your candy craving is really an unconscious need for serotonin, then snack on a whole-grain English muffin drizzled with honey or a toasted cinnamon bagel with jam.

- **Tip #12: Spice it up.** Sweet-tasting spices and flavorings, such as vanilla, cinnamon, mint and nutmeg, are calorie-free alternatives to sugar

- **Tip #13: Think produce**. Use dessert time to help meet your daily quota of eight fruits and vegetables. Have a poached pear, a baked apple, frozen blueberries or canned mandarin oranges sprinkled with candied ginger.

- **Tip #14: Change your attitude.** Sweet cravings are a suggestion to eat, not a command to pig out. You are in charge of what goes into your mouth. Any time you are tempted to reach for some junky, sugary snack, remind yourself that you deserve better.

- **Tip #15: Purchase unsweetened versions of your favorite foods, then sweeten them at home.** You won't add the amount of sugar that is in the processed version. For example, a half cup of sweetened applesauce or a packet of cinnamon-spice oatmeal each have more than 4 teaspoons of added sugar, while there is no added sugar in plain applesauce or oats. Plain yogurt only has the natural lactose found in milk, while fruited yogurts have six or more teaspoons of added sugar.

- **Tip #16: Put added sugar into perspective.** It's easy to get wound up about the sugar in processed foods. Just make sure your efforts are in the right place. Yes, there is a lot of sugar in ketchup, bottled salad dressing and barbecue sauce, but you eat these items by the teaspoon. It is the scones, muffins, cookies and other items eaten by the handful that add the most unwanted sugar.

- **Tip #17: Pamper yourself.** Your best bet for curbing sugar cravings when stressed is to never get stressed in the first place. Read a book, meditate daily, do yoga, take bubble baths, walk in the woods, romp with the dog or go for a bike ride on a regular basis before you tense up, turn to sweets and pack on the pounds. You have a choice: do you want to drink 162 calories in a cola or walk off the same amount of calories during a 35-minute stress-busting walk? Sure, you can temporarily soothe stress with the 340 calories in a slice of apple pie, but a 75-minute walk will burn the same calories and take inches off your hips.

Happy Sweets

In the mood for a little sweet thing? Here are 15 good-for-you options.

1. **Berry Lavender Parfait:** Top fresh berries or other fruit with a container of Rachel's Wickedly Delicious Plum Honey Lavender yogurt. Top with a dollop of fat-free dessert topping.

2. **Grilled Peaches:** Cut fresh peaches in half. Peel and pit, then toss with 1 teaspoon each canola oil, brandy extract and honey. Grill on the barbecue until slightly charred, about three minutes. Turn and grill until grill marks form. Serve.

3. **Pineapple Coconut Smoothie:** See recipe in the Recipes section.

4. **Rice Pudding:** Make it with brown rice, DHA-fortified low-fat milk or soy milk, egg substitute and dried fruit.

5. **Minty Ginger Melon:** Whip a teaspoon of honey, a teaspoon of mint and a teaspoon each of grated fresh ginger in a food processor. Pour over cantaloupe cubes.

6. **Mango Granita:** Blend a peeled and seeded mango, ¼ cup orange juice, juice of one small lime and a slice of fresh ginger. Pour into a bowl and freeze. Scrape frozen fruit mixture with a fork into individual serving bowls and serve.

7. **Apple Pie Apples:** Slice and seed apples. Sprinkle with cinnamon sugar.

8. **Mother Nature's Candy Bar:** Stuff each of four lemon-flavored pitted dried plums with an almond for a chewy, sweet, crunchy alternative to a candy bar.

9. **Banana Split:** Make with 2 scoops fat-free, double-churned ice cream, one banana, 1 tablespoon chopped nuts, ½ cup fresh or frozen berries and 3 tablespoons fat-free dark chocolate syrup.

10. **Sugar-free Orange Jell-O:** Make with 100% orange juice instead of water.

11. **Poached Pears in Chocolate Lavender Sauce:** See recipe in the Recipes section.

12. **Tapioca Pudding:** Make with DHA-fortified low-fat milk and top with fresh fruit.

13. **Nut Bread Spread:** Top a slice of date-nut bread with fat-free cream cheese and diced dates or figs.

14. **Fruit Ambrosia:** Mix 1 cup pineapple cubes, two sliced bananas, 1 drained can mandarin oranges, one container of Rachel's Wickedly Delicious Vanilla Chai yogurt and ¼ cup minimarshmallows. Makes four servings.

15. **Cherry Swirl Strudel Ring with Lemon Glaze:** See recipe in the Recipes section.

Avoid the Knee-Jerk Reaction

Happy, fit people pay attention, unlike some of us who give in to a craving for sweets before our conscious minds are even engaged. We stand at the kitchen counter and eat half the apple pie right out of the pan. We numb ourselves with a bag of Oreos before we even notice we've opened the bag. Happy, lean folks don't do that. Here are a few tips for avoiding this mindless eating:

1. Remember the 10-minute rule. Give yourself 10 minutes before indulging in any sweet treat. You may find that by stepping back for just a few minutes out of your entire life that it is enough to watch the crave wave crest and fall.

2. Measure your hunger. Before you dive into the ice cream, ask yourself, "On a scale of 1 to 5, just how hungry am I?" Only entertain the notion of eating if you are above a 3, which is moderately hungry. And even in those cases, make a rule that you will eat at least three healthy foods, such as an apple, a serving of leftover spaghetti and a glass of milk, before you have something sweet.

3. Eat every four to five hours. Set your watch if you are tempted to snack before the four-hour limit. If you are hungry more frequently than this, you may have chosen the wrong foods at the last meal. Pack healthy snacks, like a thermos of soy milk, 100% whole-wheat crackers, low-fat string cheese, a piece of fruit, a bag of baby carrots and/or a can of tomato juice.

4. Plan your meals. Make sure to include fiber-rich, water-packed foods, such as salads, cooked whole-grains and fruits that fill you up on few calories.

Sweet Solutions

Making a few changes in how much and when you eat sugar can do what no medication can. It can rebalance your brain chemistry and curb out-of-control appetites for a *natural high*. Better yet, it comes with no side effects other than improved energy, sharper thinking, lower risk for most age-related diseases and a longer and more fulfilling life. Happy, fit people who take good care of themselves even look 20 years younger than those who feast on the sugary and highly processed stuff. You deserve to look and feel great, so every time you start to eat anything, step back and ask yourself, "Will this food help or hurt me?" Unless a food is a step toward health and bliss, it probably is not worth the taste.

SECRET 5:
SPRINKLE IT WITH SUPER MOOD FOODS

The Promise

In one week of making this change, you will:

- have more energy
- begin to appreciate the flavor of foods

In one month, you will:

- think more clearly
- feel less stressed
- drop a few pounds
- notice an improvement in mood

In one year, you will:

- slow your brain's aging
- lower your risk for all age-related disease
- lose weight
- feel great

The first time I met Teresa, she weighed more than 350 pounds. She was a waitress at a café on the way to the coast in Oregon, and her size made it difficult for her to maneuver between the two tables and four booths crammed into the tiny restaurant. She had a beautiful face, but it was no secret she was miserable. It was an effort for her to move her body as she shuttled orders from the kitchen to the customers.

When I stopped at the café two years later, I hardly recognized Teresa. She'd lost 192 pounds and looked like a million bucks. Not only was she lean, she was radiant. That beautiful face glowed and she moved gracefully around the café like a ballroom dancer. She walked with her shoulders back and her head high. Her smile was no longer forced. She was truly happy and it showed.

When I asked her how she had lost the weight, she said,

"I started paying attention to what the skinny people were ordering. They chose spinach salads with dressing on the side. They asked for their sandwiches on whole-grain bread with no mayo. They made a meal out of the soup of the day. They drank the fresh-squeezed orange juice, not the homemade milk shakes. They had the berries in season, not the apple pie with ice cream for dessert. It dawned on me that my weight wasn't my lot in life. I was exactly the weight I should be considering the foods I ate. If I ate like those skinny people, I'd look like them."

And so she took cues from the happy, fit people who frequented her restaurant and, over the course of two years, dropped a ton of weight. She also regained her energy and confidence. She was happy, vibrant and obviously pleased with herself.

What Teresa didn't realize is that by eating like her happy, fit customers, she was following a diet based on real foods with an emphasis on some of the most powerful super mood foods Mother Nature has to offer. That diet not only helped her lose weight, but it kept her happy in the process. The next time I stopped at the café, Teresa was gone. The new waitress told me she'd fallen in love and gotten married. The last they had heard from her was a postcard from Rome.

This Time, Do It Right!

The best diet plans help you get around the deprivation issue by ensuring you get plenty of low-calorie foods so you don't go hungry—a rumbling stomach is a guaranteed road to bad-moodsville. That's a great strategy. Why not take it one step further and follow a diet trick or two from people, like Teresa, who have lost weight and stayed happy by adding a few of the tried-and-true foods known to boost mood, memory *and* drop pounds?

Yes, there are a few foods, when added to a calorie- and portion-controlled real foods diet, that can give you an added kick in the mood butt, as well as speed weight loss. They also sharpen your mind and reduce stress, which is pretty amazing, since most fad diets increase stress hormones, make us dumber, slow our reaction times, muddle the mind—and then fail in the long run.

Happy superfoods. Choose the right foods and they keep you on a steady course of feeling your best. "I see many people fall into the 'dieting depression,' which lowers motivation and undermines a person's chances at successfully losing weight, and more importantly, keeping the weight off," says John Foreyt, Ph.D., Director of the Nutrition Research Center at Baylor College of Medicine in Houston and an expert on weight management. To avoid this trap, you should set realistic goals, take little steps toward successful weight loss and sprinkle your diet with a few superfoods that nourish your mood, mind and body.

Combine what you learned in Chapter 1 about real foods with the super mood foods in this chapter and you are guaranteed to feel amazing and lose weight. That's what Whitney, a public relations executive in San Francisco, found:

> "I eat really well when I'm at home and have lots of energy and feel great. But I don't think I truly appreciated how important eating the

right foods are until my job required travel. That's when I eat the processed stuff. It makes me feel awful, fat and bloated (especially salty things), which is probably why I feel so tired when I'm on the road. Now I really get how eating right can make a world of difference in your energy and mood."

If your typical diet is like Whitney's travel fare, then you will be amazed how great you feel when you switch to a real-foods diet trimmed in super foods.

The Natural High

Eating right is not about a handful of foods, but rather the healthiness of the entire diet. That said, a few foods are truly super, packing in more than their share of nutrients and phytonutrients that boost memory, energy and mood and reduce stress, while at the same time helping guarantee permanent weight loss and tasting divine.

The Story Behind Superfoods

Lots of processed foods at the grocery store, from exotic juices to designer yogurts, try to convince you they are packed with more than their share of nutrients or antioxidants. Most are more hype than help. What truly makes a food super?

- It must have a ton of nutrients for only a few calories. Think of it as a super-low "cal-a-nut" ratio—for each calorie you get a whopping dose of waist-slimming fiber and mood-boosting vitamins and minerals.
- There must be proof that this food speeds weight loss, revs metabolism, aids in burning body fat, fills you up on fewer calories and/or helps you stick with your diet.
- It must be loaded with antioxidants. These are the nutrients and close to a million phytonutrients in unprocessed foods that protect the brain from little oxygen fragments, called free radicals, that otherwise speed aging, clog memory, dampen your mood, increase stress and even drain energy.

A food must have all these qualities to make the grade. Granted, some foods are higher in antioxidants or have a low cal-a-nut ratio, but since they don't meet the other two criteria, they fall short on being a super mood food.

Of course, there are tons of supernutritious foods that are great inclusions in any diet, but to list them all would fill volumes. So I'm picking my 12 favorites. Add these to the real foods discussed in the other chapters and you have a one-two punch for boosting mood and slimming your waistline.

What Do Free Radicals Have to Do with You?

Super mood foods are loaded with antioxidants. To understand why these are so important, you need a short course in free radicals.

Free radicals are oxygen fragments inhaled in air pollution and tobacco smoke, consumed in fatty foods and generated in the body during normal metabolic processes. Left unchecked, these oxygen fragments, or oxidants, attack cell membranes and the genetic code, a process called oxidation. Your body "rusts" when exposed to oxygen, which causes cells to either die or mutate. Cell "rusting," or oxidation, contributes to all age-related diseases, from heart disease and cancer to cataracts and possibly osteoporosis.

Free radicals also damage the delicate communication pathways in your brain. Minute by minute, day by day, year after year, decade upon decade, free radicals are attacking and damaging one brain cell after another until the buildup results in memory loss, slowed reaction times, reduced alertness and even Alzheimer's disease. The damage they do to brain cells also contributes to fatigue, feeling blue and being stressed out. Next time you walk into a room and can't remember why you came in there or once again forgot where you put your keys, you might be experiencing firsthand the effects of daily free radical attacks.

Gimme My Antioxidants

The good news is, your body has an anti–free radical system, called antioxidants, that prevents oxidants from damaging cells. Antioxidants also help keep the heart beating strong and protect the tiny blood vessels that transport nutrients and oxygen to brain cells. Since 20% of the heart's output goes to the brain, all of these benefits mean improved blood flow and better thinking, more energy, improved mood and less stress. The trick is to maintain an antioxidant arsenal equal to or better than the daily onslaught of free radicals.

Stockpiling antioxidants is essential throughout life, especially when we are stressed and as we age. Stress is a death sentence for brain cells. Feeling tense and anxious sets off a cascade of events, releasing chemicals and hormones, including cortisol, that generate a free-radical flood that is toxic to brain cells and that undermines your ability to think and be happy. No wonder people with high blood levels of cortisol score lower on memory tests compared to people who are relatively stress-free. As we get older, oxidative damage to tissues, including the brain, intensifies; that means a 60-year-old needs more antioxidant-rich foods than a 30-year-old, who needs more than a 12-year-old.

Rating the Antioxidants

All fruits and vegetables, whole grains, legumes, tea, chocolate and wine—in short, just about any real food—have antioxidants. What makes one super and one not? It's the amount of antioxidants.

To measure a food's antioxidant content, researchers use the ORAC test, which stands for Oxygen Radical Absorbance Capacity. This is a measure of the total antioxidant content in a given food and thus how many free radicals a specific food can absorb and destroy. The more oxygen radicals a food absorbs, the higher its ORAC score. The higher its ORAC score, the better it is at helping our bodies prevent memory loss and cope with stress.

Nutrition experts estimate each one of us needs a minimum of 3,000 ORAC points a day to even begin to protect the mind, mood and body, though most Americans average less than half that amount. A daily ORAC intake of 10,000 or more is even better. In fact, no one has yet found an upper limit. Most of the 12 super mood foods listed below have hearty ORAC scores.

You can't store antioxidants, so you must replenish ORAC points every day. That means you need these and lots of other real foods in just about every meal you eat.

A word of caution.

Many tests promise to evaluate your antioxidant status. They might take urine, skin or blood samples to measure by-products of free radical metabolism. Assessing antioxidant status, however, is not that simple and never gives you the whole picture of what's going on in your body. For example, one test uses a scanner that shines a laser through your finger. It measures only a handful of carotenoids, not the entire gamut of close to a million antioxidants in the fruits, vegetables and other real foods you eat. There's also a catch—the company that markets the scanner also sells supplements specifically designed to raise blood levels of the few carotenoids they are testing (surprise!). In reality, the only way to be guaranteed your antioxidant arsenal is stocked is to eat a real-foods diet with daily inclusions of some of the superfoods in this chapter.

A Word About Variety

Variety is the spice of life.

Variety is the soul of pleasure.

The joy of life is variety.

No pleasure endures unseasoned by variety.

Variety, variety, variety. You've heard the rule a million times: eat a variety of foods. Of course, those wise diet gurus aren't recommending you eat a variety of doughnuts, cookies, chips, cupcakes and other junk. No, they mean a variety of real foods—fruits, vegetables, nuts, seeds, whole grains, legumes and more. For one thing, no one food supplies all the nutrients you need. Therefore, the more varied your diet, the more likely you will get the right dose of all the 40+ nutrients.

Second, foods are not all fun and games. Even the most nutritious food contains a harmful substance or two. For example, cabbage is absolutely packed with fiber, vitamins and antioxidants. On the flip side, it also contains compounds called goitrogens that interfere with your thyroid. No big deal if you eat cabbage a few times a week, but go on some cabbage diet, feasting only on platters of cabbage day after day, and you might have a problem. Eat a variety of foods and you avoid overdosing on any one harmful substance.

Third, you get the best antioxidant protection when you eat different antioxidant-rich foods. For example, drink only mangosteen juice or limit your fruit to just handfuls of berries every day and your antioxidant levels rise, but that does not necessarily mean you'll think better or live longer. You need a variety of superfoods every day. Eat blueberries and nuts today, strawberries and oranges tomorrow, pomegranates on your spinach salad the next day and so forth, and antioxidant levels soar, plus you think better, feel better and outlive everybody.

The message here: choose a diet based on real foods, sprinkle that diet with a variety of super mood foods and vary your choices from meal to meal, day to day and week to week.

IncrEdibles: The Dynamic Dozen

From soup to nuts, the following 12 foods pack a huge mood and waist-slimming punch. Add them as often as possible to your real-food diet. Of course, many other foods are super mood foods, too. But, for the sake of space, start with these.

1. Nuts

Kristen, a nurse in Ohio, had the hardest time sticking to diets:

> "I was the classic yo-yoer. I've tried low-carb and high-carb, SlimFast and Jenny Craig, fasting and soup diets. Oh sure, all of them worked at first. I'd drop a few pounds, but then the weight came back. This is going to sound silly, but what finally worked for me was snacking on nuts. Of course, I also had to exercise and pay attention to portions like I'd done on the other diets, but just having that one moment during the day when I could have something really satisfying was enough to keep me on track. I've lost 25 pounds and kept it off for five years."

Many people are much more successful when they add a few healthy fats, such as nuts and olive oil, to their weight-loss diets than if they try to stick with very-low-fat diets. There are three reasons why nuts help you stay happy and fit.

1. Nuts are fiber-rich, so even an ounce is enough to take the edge off hunger. (Their phytonutrient and antioxidant ORAC scores are high, too. For example, an ounce of pistachios packs 2,661 ORAC points, while pecans tally a whopping 5,980 on the ORAC scale!)

2. Nuts raise the metabolic rate by up to 11%, thus helping burn more calories.

3. Nuts help regulate blood sugar. They have a low glycemic index (GI). Compared to potatoes or corn flakes, which rank in the 80s on the GI scale, peanuts and other nuts rank as low as 14, meaning they don't raise blood sugar levels and thus don't stimulate appetite or fat storage. Peanuts also contain a compound called arginine that helps regulate the hormone insulin, which helps maintain normal blood sugar levels. The more you control blood sugar, the easier time you'll have managing your weight, which explains why an ounce of nuts a day helps slim waistlines.

Speaking of peanuts, these nuts are weird. You may think of them as a nut, but they really are a bean. In fact, they straddle the fence between nuts and legumes, which is a good thing. That means they have all the good stuff of a nut, such as the healthy fats, magnesium and vitamin E, but they also have all the nutrition advantages of a bean, such as folic acid, potassium and phytonutrients (called saponins and sterols). All those nutrients improve mood, aid in sleep and/or help you better cope with stress. They even have something in common with red wine, resveratrol, an antioxidant that helps keep your arteries elastic and squeaky clean. (Unfortunately, roasting destroys resveratrol.)

How much? 1 ounce a day.

Eat more: Eat nuts plain or toss them into salads, cereals or yogurt. Add nuts to meatless stir frys or to pancake and muffin batters. Make homemade trail mix with equal parts nuts and dried fruit (such as dried tart cherries). Replace pine nuts with other nuts, such as pistachios, when making pesto sauce. Add nuts to salads or to desserts. Combine nuts with yogurt, apples and celery to make a quick Waldorf salad. Dip baby carrots in peanut butter. Coat fish or chicken with ground nuts before cooking.

2. Soy

Happy, fit people repeatedly tell me that they lost more weight when they added soy to their calorie-controlled diets than when they added other protein-rich foods, like beef or whey powders.

It could be soy's protein, since protein is much more filling than either fat or carbs. Also the protein in soy is lean, which is far superior to the greasy protein in most red meats.

What sets soy apart from other protein-rich foods, however, is that soy also has phytoestrogens, compounds that help burn body fat. The combination of protein and phytoestrogens is superpowerful for weight loss, since it helps satisfy you on fewer calories and boosts metabolism. Soy also curbs elevated blood sugar and reduces blood cholesterol and insulin levels.

Beyond weight loss, soy has superpowers in boosting memory. It might be because of the phytoestrogens, or maybe it is the antioxidants in soy that protect the brain and possibly improve mood. People who eat soy-based foods (not supplements!) show less damaging effects on brain tissue during stress, and their brains stay youthful even into their later years, which means better memory and thinking ability. And it's never too late. Memory improves at all stages of life, even into your seventies or beyond, when soy is included regularly in the diet.

How much? 25 grams of soy protein a day, or the equivalent of three glasses of soy milk.

Eat more: Use soy milk to replace milk in meals and recipes, especially brands that are fortified with the omega-3 fat DHA. Sprinkle edemame (green soybeans) in salads and side dishes. Substitute mashed tofu for ricotta cheese in recipes or add to egg dishes. Snack on dry-roasted soy nuts. Or try any of the delicious recipes with soy in this book.

3 and 4. Milk and Yogurt

It seemed a fluke when the first study reported that calcium aids weight loss; a mineral that builds bone could not possibly burn body fat.

Further studies showed as calcium intake increased, body fat decreased. With each glass of milk (or 300 milligram increase in regular calcium intake), a person could expect to lose 5 to 6 pounds of body fat. In fact, as calcium intake goes up, body fat goes down. One study comparing people consuming either very-low-calorie diets (800 calories a day), 800-calorie diets based on milk products, or 1,300-calorie diets based on milk products, found that people on the 1,300-calorie diet lost three times as much weight as those on the low-calcium 800-calorie diet. Lose more weight by eating more food? Now that's a great diet!

How does calcium help with weight loss? Although poorly understood, calcium is important in energy metabolism and especially in storing and burning body fat. High-calcium diets might help block calories from being stored as fat on your hips and thighs, thus reducing the chance of gaining weight during times of overeating. The combination of calcium and vitamin D seems to be most effective at burning fat tissue, but it is unclear exactly why. Or maybe it is a mood issue, since calcium helps to balance mood during stressful times. Here's the best part—chocolate milk has all the weight-busting potential of plain milk, plus more than 3,000 ORAC points per glass!

Yogurt is just as good, and it provides healthy bacteria to prevent bloating and help flatten the tummy. You have good and bad bacteria in your gut. The good guys, the ones in yogurt (especially *acidophilus*, *bifidum* and *rhamnosus*), help keep the gastrointestinal tract in tip-top working order and reduce gas or constipation. Stick to plain, nonfat yogurt and sweeten it yourself at home with jam or fruit.

The link with calcium and weight still needs more proof, but since calcium is needed for a host of other stuff, from building bones to taking the crankiness out of PMS, it is wise to add at least 1,000 milligrams of calcium from nonfat milk products to a daily weight-loss plan.

How much? Three cups a day of nonfat or 1% milk or two cups of yogurt.

Eat more: Cook rice or oatmeal in milk. Add milk to coffee or tea. Add nonfat dry milk powder to pancake or muffin batters. Layer fruit and yogurt in a parfait glass or make pudding with nonfat milk for desserts. Top waffles or French toast with yogurt and fruit. Make creamed soups and sauces with evaporated nonfat milk instead of cream. Use undiluted evaporated milk in mashed potatoes. Blend milk or yogurt with fruit for smoothies. Use plain yogurt instead of sour cream for dips, salad dressing and toppings; mix equal parts low-fat mayonnaise and yogurt for coleslaw or potato salad.

5. Dark Green Leafies

As a nerdy dietitian, it's difficult for me to understand how anyone can be happy without dark green leafies in the daily diet. From spinach, chard and collards to leaf lettuce, beet greens and broccoli, these are the very best sources of the B vitamin folate. Your brain cells won't turn on without it. It's no wonder that poor intake of folate increases the risk for depression, fatigue, poor memory and possibly even more serious mental problems like schizophrenia. People battling the blues who boost their intake of greens say they feel better and happier as a result. (Remember, it was spinach salads, not iceberg salads, that those happy, fit people at Teresa's café were eating.) People who are clinically depressed only respond to antidepressant therapy if their blood levels of folate are high.

Packed with vitamins and minerals, one serving of dark greens supplies an entire day's requirement for vitamin A, more than 3 milligrams of iron, almost a third of your daily need for folate, and hefty amounts of calcium and B vitamins, all for about 20 calories. A one-cup serving of cooked Swiss chard supplies more than half of a woman's daily recommendation for magnesium, a mineral that helps her cope with stress, curbs symptoms of PMS and aids in sleep. Phytonutrients, such as sulforaphane in broccoli and the carotenoids in carrots, spinach or romaine lettuce, clear toxins from the body and strengthen your resistance to colds and infections. On top of that, a cup of broccoli adds 3,632 ORAC points and a cup of raw spinach adds another 4,040 ORAC points to the daily menu.

How much? Two servings a day (one serving is 1 cup raw or ½ cup cooked).

Eat more: Replace iceberg lettuce in salads and sandwiches with leaf lettuce or spinach; layer greens into lasagna; use large spinach leaves instead of a tortilla to wrap around cheese, beans and salsa. Lightly steam chopped collards and mix into mashed potatoes. Add greens to stir-frys, soups and stews. Sauté them in a little olive oil and garlic.

6. Dark Orange Vegetables

"I feel so much better when I snack on carrots and peanut butter than when I pig out on chips and other greasy foods," says Lana, a waitress in San Diego who has lost 15 pounds in the past year. Maybe it's the crunch. Or maybe it's the fiber. Then again, even a small serving of deep-orange vegetables supplies five times the Daily Value for beta-carotene, an antioxidant that protects the brain from damage. The more richly colored vegetables you eat, the more brain protection you get. Bright orange veggies also supply hefty amounts of vitamin C, potassium and iron and more fiber than a slice of whole-wheat bread or a bowl of oatmeal. For every half-cup serving, their ORAC scores range from 528 for butternut squash and 884 for carrots to 2,820 for sweet potatoes.

Besides, the more colorful fruits and vegetables you eat, the sharper your mind and the easier it is to lose weight and keep it off. The more produce you include in your daily diet and the longer you eat that way, the longer you will live healthy and the sharper your mind.

How much? 1+ cup a day.

Eat more: Microwave and top sweet potatoes with maple syrup and pecans. Puree cooked yams or carrots and add to soups as a thickener. Use sweet potatoes instead of potatoes in salads. Slice sweet potatoes into wedges, salt and bake at 425 degrees for 15 minutes for golden fries. Cook, mash and use winter squash instead of noodles or rice as a base for any dish. Add roasted butternut squash cubes to canned soups.

More Produce, Less Pesticides

To minimize pesticides in your diet:

- Wash and scrub all fresh fruits and vegetables, especially the worst offenders, such as apples and bell peppers.
- Soak tender produce, such as berries.
- Peel fruits or vegetables when possible, especially the worst offenders, such as peaches.
- Discard outer leaves of leafy vegetables, such as romaine lettuce.

- Eat a variety of produce to minimize your exposure to any one pesticide.
- Buy local. Shop at the farmer's market where produce is less likely to be sprayed.

7. Broth Soups

The ultimate trick to permanent weight loss is to feel satisfied on fewer calories. That trick includes two accomplices: fiber and water.

We all push back from the table when we have eaten a given weight of food, according to research from the Pennsylvania State University. Since a pound of celery supplies fewer calories than a pound of chocolate, it's no surprise that happy, fit people who design their diets around fiber- and water-packed foods, such as vegetables, soups, stews and smoothies, fill up on fewer calories, feel satisfied between meals and have an easier time managing their weights compared to those who snack on chips and cookies.

People average about 135 calories less when the meal contains soup. That might not sound like much, but over the course of a year it equates to a 14-pound loss! Weight-loss experts predict that if Americans cut just 100 calories a day, it would halt the obesity epidemic in this country. That's three bites of food, 10 minutes of walking or a daily bowl of soup.

That's exactly what Jennifer, an accountant in Chicago, found when she switched from a bag to a thermos for lunch:

> "I have a desk job, which means it is easy for me to gain weight if I'm not careful about what I eat. I was gaining slowly, but surely, for the last couple of years even though I brought my own lunch and tried to make it healthy. When I switched to a thermos of soup, a yogurt and a piece of fruit for lunch, I found that it filled me up and kept me going through the afternoon and I wasn't as tempted to grab a piece of chocolate off a coworker's desk."

The trick is to make calorie-dilute foods, such as broth-based soups, stews, smoothies, and fruits and vegetables (other than fried potatoes) the basis of a meal plan, not the whole diet. To boost the ORAC score, the soup should be loaded with colorful vegetables, such as carrots, green peas, sweet potato chunks and spinach. (Hint: soup-only diets don't work, but soup added to a healthful diet does.)

How much? Serve a broth-based soup for one meal (lunch or dinner) on most days.

Eat more: Make a big batch of homemade vegetable soup to use throughout the week. Season with Mrs. Dash or True Lemon to make the flavor pop without salt. Use canned soups with the word *healthy* in the title and add extra frozen peas and carrots or chopped spinach. At restaurants, make soup your main course.

8. Legumes

We all know that beans are mind-bogglingly good for you. Whether they are lentils, chick peas, split peas or black, kidney, navy or pinto beans, legumes are packed with nutrients that improve mood, such as folate, calcium, copper, magnesium, iron and zinc. The folate in beans protects against a memory-destroying compound called homocysteine. The antioxidant phytonutrients in legumes, such as saponins and phytosterols, lower cancer and heart disease risk. Their massive antioxidant content explains why their ORAC scores are so high: a cup of beans has between 4,000 and 13,000 ORAC points!

Beans are the perfect diet food. They are almost fat-free but high in protein, water and fiber—the magic combo for feeling full and satisfied on few calories. One cup of cooked legumes has up to 16 grams of fiber! You would have to eat eight slices of whole-wheat bread, five bananas or four cups of corn to get that much fiber. Legumes are very low on the glycemic index and thus help regulate blood sugar as well as appetite.

Yet, bean cuisine is low on people's priority lists— most of us average only about a cup of beans a *year*, a pittance compared to the 50 pounds of pork we gobble at the same time.

It is hard to get excited about "the musical fruit," no matter how nutritious, tasty and antioxidant-packed it is. That is, until you start listing specifics. "If I tell my family we are having beans for dinner, all I get is a chorus of moans," says Eleanor, a working mom in Cincinnati. "But if I tell them we are having Boston baked beans with corn bread or creamy lentil soup with chipotle sauce, their mouths start to water." So get the frown off your face and start looking for excuses to add more beans to your diet—your mood and waistline will thank you for it.

How much? One cup at least four times a week.

Eat more: Use beans in salads and burritos, or sprinkle with cilantro and serve hot on top of rice. Add extra canned beans to soups. Skip the ranch dip and dunk vegetables in hummus.

Degassing Beans

The offending substances in beans that cause bloating and gas are a special type of starch. People who don't eat beans frequently have low levels of the enzyme that breaks down this starch, so bacteria in the gut do it for them, with the unpopular side effect of gas. The good news: the more beans you eat, the less likely you will suffer from gas, since your body will make more of that important enzyme. In the meantime, to degas beans:

- Soak raw beans, then discard the water before cooking.
- Cook beans thoroughly.
- Eat slowly, so you don't gulp air, which only worsens the problem.
- Use Beano, which supplies the enzyme your body is missing.
- Drink lots of water.
- For canned beans, drain liquid and rinse beans.

9. Citrus

Sweet and tart, fresh and clean. If morning sunshine had a scent it would be citrus; that aroma also holds the secret to a happy mood and weight loss.

Citrus fruit is one of the most nutritious of all the fruits. A cup of grapefruit sections supplies 1,104 ORAC points and your entire day's requirement for vitamin C. A glass of OJ supplies 165% of a woman's RDA for vitamin C and 1,936 ORAC points (that's because it takes about a pound of oranges to make a cup of OJ).

Moodwise, vitamin C is important in boosting energy, since it helps absorb iron and maintain healthy red blood cells that carry oxygen to every cell in the body, including the brain. Without iron, your brain literally suffocates, leaving you groggy, depressed, too pooped to appreciate life and totally unmotivated. The vitamin C in citrus also helps curb the stress response, lowering stress hormone levels and possibly reducing blood pressure. People even report they feel calmer during stress when they consume enough vitamin C.

Oranges are brimming with folate (a B vitamin essential to brain function and mood), while all citrus are overflowing in phytonutrients, fiber and potassium, a mineral essential for energy and preventing fatigue. Just 1 cup of any citrus juice supplies about a quarter of your daily potassium needs (you'd have to drink twice as much apple juice to get the same amount of potassium). Hundreds of different phytonutrients have been identified in citrus, with names like terpenes, flavonoids, coumarins and carotenoids. Most of these phytonutrients protect the brain and improve memory.

How much? 1+ serving a day (one piece of fruit or a 6-ounce glass of juice).

Eat more: Oranges are the perfect bring-along snack. Or place a bowl of grapefruit sections on the dining table or at your work desk. Make fruit smoothies or parfaits with oranges. Mix orange sections into yogurt. Dunk orange sections in fat-free dark chocolate syrup. In recipes, pair oranges or grapefruit with roasted sweet potatoes in a salad, use fresh orange or lime juice and maple syrup for marinades, and mix orange sections into guacamole, tossed salads and rice dishes. Add lemon juice or zest to any dish to enhance flavor.

10. Wheat Germ

You don't get much better on the cal-a-nut ratio than with wheat germ. The heart of the wheat kernel is a gold mine of nutrition. Half a cup of toasted wheat germ supplies 100% of your daily need for folic acid and 50% of your magnesium, zinc and vitamin E requirements. Vitamin E–rich diets help prevent and slow the progression of—and might even lower the risk for developing—Alzheimer's disease by up to 70%. Wheat germ supplies decent amounts of trace minerals, such as iron and zinc. You also get a truckload of phytonutrients, including octacosanol, a compound that improves endurance and helps the body cope with stress.

How much? ¼ cup or more a day.

Eat more: Sprinkle on oatmeal or yogurt, add to cookie and pancake batters, mix into muffin or meatloaf recipes or blend with honey and peanut butter for a sandwich spread.

11. Tart Cherries

You know they make a great pie, but you might not know that this ruby-red fruit is a rich source of a wide array of nutrients, including fiber, potassium, magnesium, iron, vitamin A, vitamin C, vitamin B_6, vitamin E and folate. They have a low-glycemic index score of 54 (any score less than 55 is considered low), thus producing a mild rise in blood sugar levels associated with lowered risks for diabetes and weight gain.

Just slightly more than 3 ounces of tart cherry juice concentrate supplies 12,800 ORAC points (that's because there are 100 fresh cherries in an 8-ounce glass of cherry juice). A quarter cup of dried cherries rates 3,060 on the ORAC scale. In fact, a study from the University of Minnesota found that cherries, with their high amount of anthocyanins, were in the top 33 foods for highest antioxidant content, surpassing well-known leaders, such as red wine, prunes and dark chocolate. These anthocyanins protect brain cells from oxidative damage associated with nerve damage, thus lowering the risk for memory loss, dementia and even Alzheimer's disease. They might even help reverse brain aging. (While tart cherries are rich sources of anthocyanins, maraschino cherries are not, since the delicate phytochemical is lost in the processing and replaced with food coloring.)

Finally, cherries might be useful for both sleep and memory. They are one of the few foods that contain melatonin, a hormone that helps regulate sleep. A few studies also show that the anthocyanins in cherries might aid with weight loss.

How much? One cup of raw tart cherries or a ¼ cup of dried tart cherries four times a week.

Eat more: Add dried tart cherries to side dishes, such as rice pilafs or vegetable dishes. Mix dried tart cherries with peanut butter for a new twist on the PB & J, add cherries to oatmeal cookie recipes in place of raisins, and toss in dried cherries when making apple pie. Add dried tart cherries to tossed salads, fruit salads and slaws. Include dried tart cherries in baked items. Use tart cherry juice in smoothies, toddies, iced teas, punches, lemonades, sangrias and coolers.

12. Berries

Gladys attributes her sharp-as-a-tack 98-year-old memory to the berries she has eaten all her life. "As a kid raised on a farm in southern Oregon, my sisters and I used to sneak off after dinner and have our dessert standing in the berry patch eating right off the vine," she recalls. Gladys never lost her love of berries and still eats them every day. "I hold my own at Jeopardy, which isn't bad for someone my age, especially since I'm up against my great-grandchildren!"

These sweet and juicy fruits are the perfect water and fiber combination for weight loss. They also are loaded with B vitamins, vitamin C and antioxidants, such as flavonoids, resveratrol and more than 40 different anthocyanins. In fact, a cup of berries adds anywhere from 6,000 to 13,000 ORAC points to the daily diet. These potent antioxidants strengthen tissue defenses against oxidation and inflammation, which are underlying factors in most age-related diseases, from heart disease and cancer to memory loss, Parkinson's and Alzheimer's. The antioxidants in berries might even help reverse memory loss. Best of all, frozen berries are just as antioxidant-packed as fresh, so enjoy these nutrient gold mines all year around.

Berries are more than just antioxidants. Research from Tufts University shows that these little fruits regulate our genes! They turn on the cells' production of disease-fighting chemicals that then work 24/7 to protect the brain and all the body's tissues from damage. No wonder they improve cell communication, stimulate nerve cell growth and enhance brain cell connections. Wow!

How much? One or more cups of berries three times a week.

Eat more: Switch from ice cream to frozen blueberries for an after-dinner snack. Blend into smoothies or add to homemade salsa. Dip strawberries in fat-free chocolate syrup. Layer with yogurt for a parfait. Add to tossed salads or muffin and pancake batters. Briefly cook blueberries with a little Splenda, lemon juice and corn starch and use as a topping for pancakes, French toast, waffles and ice cream.

Anti-Superfoods: Avoid at All Costs!

- **Salad dressing:** A plate of crispy greens is one of life's little fat-free pleasures. But many fatty concoctions are guzzled under the guise of salad fixings. Salad dressing is the number one source of fat in women's diets. Drowning greens in dressing attests to the confusion over what is really a healthful salad and what is a fat-laden disaster. For example, a Grilled Chicken Caesar Salad at McDonalds has only 210 calories and almost 2 teaspoons of fat, but add a packet of dressing and you crank the calories up to 400 and the fat to more than 6 teaspoons.

  Eat less: Choose small amounts of low-fat dressings, salad spritzers or fat-free dressings. At restaurants, ask for the dressing on the side, and lightly dip the fork into the dressing and then into the salad, leaving most of the dressing behind at the end of the meal.

- **Potatoes:** One third of our daily vegetable choices are potatoes, particularly potato chips and French fries. Just 10 French fries add 158 calories and more than 2 teaspoons of fat to the diet, much of which is artery-clogging saturated or trans fats. Potatoes rank so high on the glycemic index scale that some experts say they should be placed at the top of the Food Pyramid along with sugar and fat.

  Eat less: Switch to sweet potatoes and you'll get four times the calcium and vitamin B2 and twice the vitamin C. While traditional potatoes have no beta-carotene, even a small sweet potato packs in three times your daily allotment of this potent antioxidant, which lowers your risk for heart disease and cancer and reduces the redness and skin inflammation of sunburn—a sign of accelerated aging and cancer of the skin.

- **Cheese:** We've cut back on whole milk in an effort to reduce saturated fat, but we've more than made up the difference by gobbling three times as much cheese. Cheese now outranks meat as the number one source of saturated fat in the diet. Two-thirds of that cheese is added to fast and processed foods.

  Eat less: Switch to low-fat cheeses. At restaurants, ask for half or no cheese on menu items.

- **Cream:** Between 1985 and 2001, average consumption of cream products, including sour cream, doubled to 20 half pints a person a year. It's likely intake is even higher now because of the low-carb diet fad that drove people to higher-fat fare. Cream consumption has been on a steady rise since the early 1990s, with adults today averaging more than 10 pounds of cream every year. We polish off about a half quart of ice cream every week, with a typical adult in the Midwest topping the charts at almost 42 quarts a year!

  Eat less: Fat-free half & half could save you several hundred calories a day. Switch to sorbets and low-fat ice cream (or frozen blueberries!), and keep the serving to the recommended ½ cup.

Pile It On!

If I told you I had a pill that would take 20 years off your age, help you lose weight, improve your mind and concentration, boost your mood, have all the energy you need or want, and sleep and handle stress better, would you take it? Of course you would.

Well, it isn't a pill, it's a plate. Fill your plate with piles of super mood foods and you will look, act, feel, think and sleep better. You will be leaner and healthier, too.

SECRET 6:
EMBRACE THE GOOD FAT

The Promise

In three weeks of making this change, you will:

- notice improvements in memory, reaction times and thinking ability
- possibly notice positive changes in your mood and emotions
- show a drop in cholesterol levels and risk factors for heart disease

In six months, you will:

- notice continued improvements in memory and mental function
- feel more hopeful and experience more even, positive moods throughout the day
- possibly drop a pound or two

In one year, you will:

- remember where you put your keys, the dog's name and the title of that movie
- feel more yourself, happier and calmer or less agitated
- be able to cope better than you did a year ago
- have dropped a few more pounds

Twenty years from now, you will:

- think more clearly and remember more than your friends

I make sure to get my fair share of DHA every day. I encourage my kids to take it. I caution all pregnant women to absolutely make sure they get enough of it. And every time a client complains of feeling down in the dumps or is concerned about memory problems, DHA is the first nutrient I recommend. This little fat is the most outstanding brain-boosting nutrient around. Everyone from babies to grandparents should include it in their daily diets.

Hey There, Fathead

Second only to those rolls of pudge around our waists and elsewhere, brain tissue has the most fat of any other tissue in our bodies. About 60% of our brain is fat. No, it's not stored in big bulges; in the brain, fat is a building material. Each of our 100 billion brain cells is encased, like a balloon, by a sheath or membrane made up of two layers of fat. Through that membrane, the cell gets rid of toxins, takes up nutrients and sends and receives messages.

The more fluid or flexible those fatty membranes, the better they relay and transport information. The less flexible, the more our thought processes are jammed and mood plummets. The next time you can't remember your PIN for your bank card or where you left your glasses (car keys, wallet, wedding ring...), there is a good chance the message got stuck getting through a cell membrane in your brain.

The omega-3 fats are especially flexible. That's why the brain loves them. While the grease in a hot dog or an order of carne asada goes to your hips as storage fat, the omega-3 fats are structural fats that go straight to tissues, like the brain, to keep them running in tip-top order. They make up a huge portion of the fatty membranes of brain cells and one in particular, docohexaenoic acid (DHA) accounts for 75% of the omega-3 fats in brain and nerve tissue. The more DHA you eat, the more it is incorporated into brain cells, the more flexible your brain cell membranes become, and the better, faster and more cleverly you think.

Fats 101: Omega-6s versus Omega-3s

Let's say you don't eat a lot of DHA-rich foods, but instead, like most Americans, love vegetable oils, which contain omega-6 fats. These include almost all commercial salad dressings and soy, safflower, corn or sunflower oils. You also get a truckload of these omega-6 fats in fried foods like chips, doughnuts or any food prepared in those fats, from French fries to Chicken McNuggets. Without ample DHA, the brain is forced to turn to the next best option, which are the omega-6 fats. These fats aren't as flexible, so the membranes they help build are stiffer and less efficient at moving messages, nutrients and toxins in and out of the cells.

The end result? You don't think as fast or as clearly, or remember as well. You also are more likely to feel grumpy or depressed, since stiff membranes don't manage the mood-boosting nerve chemical, serotonin, as well as the omega-3s, so serotonin gets backed up at the ends of nerve cells rather than relaying its message to be happy. That's why getting enough DHA and cutting back on vegetable oils is something happy, fit people take very seriously.

The Natural High

The more of the omega-3 fat DHA you eat, the more it is incorporated into brain cells, the more flexible your brain cell membranes become, and the better you think, the more you remember and the happier you are.

The Pollyanna Nutrient

It is a no-brainer that the omega-3 fats lower heart disease—researchers have known that for decades. Hundreds of studies, from prestigious groups like the National Institutes of Health and universities like Harvard and Tufts, repeatedly and consistently show that when you add omega-3–rich foods or supplements to the diet

- blood cholesterol and triglyceride levels drop and the good cholesterol, called HDL, goes up;

- the bad cholesterol, called LDL, changes in size so it is less harmful to arteries;
- your blood is less likely to form nasty blood clots that block arteries and lead to heart attack and stroke;
- there is less inflammation in your arteries, so they are more resistant to the development of atherosclerosis, the underlying cause of heart disease; and
- even your blood pressure and heart rate drop.

Benefits are seen whether you take omega-3s in general or only the omega-3 DHA. These benefits are experienced by men and women with heart disease, by healthy people, by vegetarians and by people at any age from infancy to the elder years. The benefits to your heart also appear to be cumulative. The more you eat, the healthier your heart. Eat omega-3–rich foods once or twice a week and you lower heart disease risk by 30%, but include those foods every day and your risk drops by up to 83%!

For years, nutrition experts focused on this exciting heart disease connection. Then a few researchers started to ponder the effects omega-3s might have on the brain. They had noticed an interesting phenomenon: people with heart disease also had an unusually high rate of depression. Could there be a common factor underlying both problems? If DHA and other omega-3 fats could dramatically lower heart disease risk, what were the possibilities for brain tissue, which is so much more dependent on these fats? DHA was the omega-3 of choice for their studies, since both the brain and the retina of the eyes contain up to 30 times more DHA than any other omega-3. There had to be a connection between those high tissue levels and DHA somehow regulating mood, memory and brain health.

In the 1990s, the results of those studies started rolling in. Study after study showed that people who are depressed and women with postpartum depression have much lower DHA levels in their blood, fat tissues and cerebrospinal fluids, up to 36% lower than happy people. It is now clear that as DHA levels drop, so do levels of the feel-good brain chemical serotonin, leaving people grumpy, blue and downright depressed. Even the severity of depression is affected; as tissue levels of omega-3s drop, depression worsens. On the other hand, boost intake of DHA by including more DHA-rich foods or by taking supplements, and serotonin levels rise and mood improves in men, women and new moms. "Studies show up to a 50% reduction in depression in people who are the toughest to treat and even an improvement in well-being for those battling everyday blues," says Joseph Hibbeln, M.D. at the National Institute for Alcohol Abuse and Alcoholism in Bethesda, Maryland.

The time factor varies from person to person; some people report improvements in mood within days or even hours of eating daily omega-3–rich meals. And it doesn't take huge amounts. Even a slight increase in blood levels, say a 1% to 5% increase, is enough to see the sneering wicked witch turn into happy-go-lucky Pollyanna.

The mood-boosting benefits of DHA go far beyond just a few studies. DHA can change the mood of entire countries. Depression rates vary up to sixty-fold from one country to another. Those rates mirror rates for heart disease and also reflect omega-3 intake. For example, as people switch from their culture's traditional diets that are adequate in omega-3s to Western-style diets almost devoid of omega-3s, the country's rates of heart disease, depression and postpartum depression skyrocket.

From Tantrums to SAD

There is more to the story than just depression and postpartum depression. Omega-3s help curb symptoms of manic depression or bipolar disease, schizophrenia and self-harm disorders, from cutting to suicide. Researchers at Purdue University found that children with low omega-3 levels are most likely to throw tantrums, have sleep problems and battle learning disabilities, while kids who are optimally nourished in these fats are least prone to attention deficit disorders. Even convicts in prison are less aggressive and angry when they take omega-3 supplements.

People who suffer from winter blues, or seasonal affective disorder (SAD), battle mild to serious depression from late fall to early spring. Typically, SAD has been linked to lack of sunlight. But studies show that even in some northern climates, like Iceland, where the dark days of winter can be pretty grim, depression rates are at an all-planet low. How do people living in gloomy climates like Iceland stay happy? Icelanders might not see much sunlight, but they eat more omega-3–rich foods, particularly fish (up to 225 pounds of seafood per person per year), than almost any other group of people on the planet. Apparently, a DHA-rich diet can reduce, if not eliminate, winter blues even when the days are long, dark and dreary.

The evidence is so overwhelming in favor of the omega-3s in the prevention and treatment of depression and mood disorders that DHA is often recommended along with antidepressant medications. The American Psychiatric Association in 2006 released a statement that the omega-3s were important when treating depression, and evidence now suggests that because omega-3s reduce anger and anxiety, they might be useful in drug and alcohol treatments. In fact, many experts suspect that depression and feelings of despair are actually good indicators or symptoms of a DHA deficiency!

No wonder this is the most amazing nutrient when it comes to staying happy.

Some Fats Are Just Plain Wrong

The more than one million Americans who slip into mild memory loss and the half a million who develop more serious dementias each year would do well to consider cutting way back on artery-clogging saturated fat and upping their DHA intake.

People who indulge in plates of artery-clogging saturated fat have flabby brains. This bad fat clogs arteries that supply oxygen to the brain, which handicaps mind power. One study from the University of California, Los Angeles found a diet high in saturated fats and sugar actually changed brain structure and reduced learning ability. In contrast, happy people who choose DHA-rich diets are the ones most likely to think clearly well into their eighties and beyond.

Why Your Memory Loves DHA

The omega-3s are critical for building and maintaining brain and nerve cells and in helping them function well. These fats give a boost to nerve chemicals, reduce inflammation, build better cell membranes and keep brain cells functioning like new. When DHA levels are low, the brain takes a nose-dive toward premature aging. Inflammation around nerves increases, brain cell membranes can't regenerate, areas of the brain that are important for memory actually shrink, and risks for serious brain and nerve disorders escalate, from Parkinson's, schizophrenia, attention deficit disorders and multiple sclerosis to dementia and Alzheimer's disease. In contrast, people who maintain high DHA levels also are the ones who protect their minds, memories and problem-solving abilities throughout life. Also, the risk for developing Alzheimer's even drops by as much as 60%! They also sleep better and cope more soundly with stress.

Avoiding Alzheimer's

My mother developed this horrible disease years ago. Thank heavens for my family's well-developed sense of humor, because that was one of the main crutches that helped us get through the 10-year process of watching our loved one disappear. I've followed the research closely, looking for any edge that might save me—and my children who would be forced to care for me—from the same fate. DHA is the most promising dietary aid I've found so far.

One of the contributing factors in Alzheimer's is the accumulation of nerve tangles, called amyloid plaque, in the brain. Preliminary research shows that DHA might help prevent these tangles by up to 40%. DHA also improves cell-to-cell communication, nerve chemical release and nerve conduction, all of which allow brain cells to effectively send messages to each other. A study from the Rush Institute for Aging in Chicago compared the dietary habits of 800 men and women between the ages of 65 and 94 years old. They found that those who included omega-3s in their weekly diets were significantly less likely to develop Alzheimer's compared to those who consumed few or no omega-3s. Now you know why I make sure to get enough DHA every day!

DHA for Kids

DHA isn't just a feel-good nutrient for grown-ups. It is critical for brain and vision development in babies and children, too. Babies born to moms who consume ample DHA during their pregnancies and while breast-feeding score higher on IQ tests later in life and have better hand-eye coordination and better vision compared to babies who didn't get enough of this critical nutrient. Those brain benefits last a lifetime.

Mothers who choose to breast-feed must make sure to get enough DHA in their diets. For mothers who don't breast-feed, it is critical that they give their babies formulas fortified with DHA, such as Enfamil Lipil, Similac Advance, Nestlé Good Start Supreme, Parent's Choice Organic, or Earth's Best with DHA.

A Stone Age Wake-up Call

Stone Age diets were based on vegetables, roots, fruits, nuts and wild game. Anthropologists estimate that the diets of our prehistoric ancestors averaged about 2,000 milligrams or more of omega-3s a day. Lucky for them, vegetable oils hadn't been invented yet, so the ratio of omega-6 to omega-3 fats was very low, or about two to one.

The omega-3 content of those diets was a key factor in our ancestors' evolution. Many experts believe that the omega-3s were important in helping our ancient ancestors develop their unique and complex nervous systems, which we inherited. For example, our ancestors' brains increased threefold in size at the same time that those ultra-great-grandparents started eating more omega-3-rich foods. Fast-forward to the present, and perhaps we can thank the omega-3s for all modern conveniences, from bagged lettuce to rocket science!

Today, few of us eat much wild game or many omega-3-rich greens, and often the only seafood to make it on the plate is a fish stick, so the average omega-3 intake has dwindled to about 100 milligrams a day—5% of what our Stone Age ancestors ate. With the glut of fried, fast-food, processed and snack items we consume, the omega-6 to omega-3 ratio now averages 11 times (some estimates are as high as 40 times) more omega-6s than omega-3s, not the two to one ratio on which humans evolved. Our bodies evolved and require omega-3s, but we can't make them. They must come from the diet.

Our totally out-of-whack ratio of omega-6 to omega-3s is the fast track to inflammation and disease in the body, including today's epidemic of heart disease, cancer, depression, attention deficit disorders, suicide, memory loss, asthma and even possibly the aggravated symptoms of premenstrual syndrome (PMS) and menopause. As omega-3 fat intake has gone down in the past few hundred years, human brain size also has started to shrink!

The Skinny on Omega-3s

Omega-3s can make you happy, but can they make you skinny? Possibly. In a handful of studies, people or animals lost more weight when the diet contained omega-3s than when it was only calorie controlled. It appears that these fats help curb hunger for hours after a meal, which any dieter will tell you is a huge factor in whether or not you stick with the plan. How the omega-3s encourage weight loss is not clear, but a few studies found that DHA inhibits fat cells from expanding and also helps regulate leptin, a hormone that tells your body how much fat to store.

Not All Omega-3s Are Created Equal

You can get all the omega-3 fat you want from flax-seeds, walnuts, canola oil, leafy greens or soy to help lower your risk for heart disease, but those foods will do nothing for your mood or memory. That's because there are three omega-3 fats, and they are not all created equal when it comes to health benefits.

The omega-3 fat in plants—from flax to walnuts—is called ALA, which stands for alpha-linolenic acid. This omega-3 shows promise in lowering heart disease risk, but that's about it. Granted, the body can convert ALA to other omega-3 fats, but the conversion is poor. One 2008 study found that eating flax was completely useless in raising levels of the other two omega-3s, EPA and DHA. Keep taking ALA-rich foods if all you want is a healthy heart. But if your goals are also to feel great, think fast and stay mentally sharp at age 100, then you won't get there with the omega-3 fat ALA.

The other two omega-3s are EPA (eicosapentaenoic acid) and DHA. These are the big guns when it comes to the omega-3s, and, even then, DHA is by far the most powerful. And since DHA can be converted to EPA in the body, you get two for one in that omega-3.

Prozac from the Sea

Fatty fish is the best dietary source of DHA and EPA. Ounce for ounce, you get the biggest omega-3 bang for your buck with salmon, herring, lake trout, anchovies and sardines. Other seafood is better than a pork chop but has considerably less of these mood- and mind-boosting fats. All the research on omega-3s and mood has used either seafood or supplements; both work equally well at keeping people happy and smart.

Your mood and mind go up and down with how much fish you eat. Eat fatty fish twice a week and you reduce the risk for developing memory loss by 28%, according to a study from Tufts. On the other hand, eat it less than once a week and depression risk goes up 34%.

Net Worth

Not all seafood is good for you. While wild salmon is rich in EPA and DHA, a white-meat fish called tilapia, a farmed fish rapidly gaining in popularity, is low in omega-3s and high in both omega-6 and saturated fats. Catfish is not much better. In other words, these fish potentially increase inflammation, which is bad for your mind and your mood. They don't count toward your goal of two servings of fish a week.

A study from the University of Kuopio in Finland found that older folks who eat fish three or more times a week significantly lower their risks for silent brain damage that otherwise contributes to stroke and dementia. In the study, people who ate the most baked or broiled fish each week were less likely to show "silent" brain infarcts, or tiny areas of tissue that have died because of insufficient blood supply, much like undetected ministrokes. However, fried fish did not produce the same benefits, possibly because fish burgers and fish sticks typically are made from fish low in the omega-3 fats and because adding omega-6 fats from oil for frying offsets the ratio of omega-6s to omega-3s and negates all the benefits of the omega-3s.

If you get your omega-3s from fish, make sure to bake, broil or poach it. Examples of great ways to get your omega-3s from the sea are found in the Recipes section of this book.

DHA or Mercury: The Fish Dilemma

The more fatty fish you eat, the more DHA you get, with conservative recommendations suggesting we need at least two servings of fatty fish a week. But here comes the dilemma: fish also is one of the most concentrated sources of mercury, a metal that is toxic to nerve cells. The more mercury you eat, the lower your brain function.

In a study from the California Pacific Medical Center in San Francisco, where fish intake was assessed in a group of men, women and children, about one in five participants warranted testing for mercury either because of high intakes of fish or because they were showing signs of mercury poisoning (i.e., fatigue, reduced memory and/or joint pain). Results showed that the mercury level for all women was 10 times that found in the general public, and some children had more than 40 times the national average. Almost all participants had blood mercury levels above 5 micrograms per liter, the maximum level recommended by the U.S. Environmental Protection Agency (EPA). Up to 18% had levels greater than 20 micrograms per liter. People with the highest mercury levels also reported eating greater amounts of swordfish, ahi and other fish known to be high in mercury.

Fortunately, these dangerously high mercury levels were reversible, although it took almost ten months to reach acceptable levels and required stopping or greatly reducing consumption of fish. The findings were so shocking that the researchers recommend that questions regarding fish consumption should be part of all comprehensive health screenings. The results of this study and others confirm that the more fish you eat, the more likely you are to consume too much mercury.

You need fish to get your DHA, but that same fish also supplies a nerve-damaging metal. One way to get around the mercury problem is to choose fish that are lower in this toxic metal, such as salmon and canned light tuna. One study even found that these high-DHA fish help block the damaging effects from mercury on the nervous system. White-meat fish, such as cod, halibut or haddock, are relatively low in mercury but also have little of those mood-boosting omega-3s. So you don't get much benefit or harm from eating them. Definitely stay away from the biggest mercury offenders, such as swordfish, albacore or ahi tuna, shark, mackerel and tilefish. Or look for foods that are fortified with DHA.

For an up-to-date guide to safe seafood, go to www.seafoodwatch.org.

Shopping for Omega-3s

If you don't like or can't afford fish, if you are vegetarian, or if you are concerned about the mercury issue in seafood, then look elsewhere in the grocery store to find your omega-3 DHA. Many foods are fortified with this healthy fat. But beware. As mentioned above, not all omega-3s are created equal. If a food is fortified with the omega-3 fat ALA, then you won't get the mood and memory boost you are hoping for. Instead, look for foods fortified with an algae-based, vegetarian source of DHA, sometimes identified as "life's DHA" on the label.

You might say "ick" at first to the thought of eating algae, but this contaminant-free source of DHA is exactly the same place fish get their omega-3s. Studies show this plant-based source of DHA is just as effective to your mental and emotional health as the DHA consumed in a salmon fillet, but without the mercury or pesticides.

A Sampling of Foods Fortified with DHA

- Bellybar nutrition bars, shakes and chews
- Most infant formulas (check labels)
- Beech-Nut® DHA plus Baby Food
- Stremick's Heritage Foods Little Einstein's Milk with DHA
- Silk soy milk Plus DHA
- Minute Maid® Enhanced Pomegranate Blueberry Juice
- Soy on the Go™ soy milk
- Rachel's Wickedly Delicious® Yogurt

- Gold Circle Farms® Eggs
- Fujisan Sushi
- Cabot 50% Reduced Fat Cheddar Cheese with DH
- Oroweat 9 Grain Bread with DHA
- Mission Life Balance Flour Tortillas
- Healthy 10™ Kefir beverage
- Crisco® Puritan® Canola Oil with Omega-3 DHA
- Pompeian OlivExtra® Plus

How Much Do You Need?

Most people are not consuming anywhere near enough DHA, but how much is optimal depends on who you talk to. The recommendations range from as little as 200 milligrams of DHA to 3.5 grams of a combination of DHA and EPA a day. Up to 1000 milligrams of DHA is used in research studies to lower heart disease

risk. Even the most conservative nutrition groups recommend at least 500 milligrams of a combination of
EPA and DHA, while you get up to a 50% reduction
in grumpy moods if you double that to 1 gram a day.
You'll get some benefits from any increase in these
fats.

Of course, it also depends on who you are and what
you eat. People who wolf down tons of omega-6 fats
really mess up their metabolism and increase their
need for the omega-3s. Ideally, those people should
cut back on vegetable oils while increasing their DHA
intakes. If they refuse to give up the fast and convenience foods, then their requirement for omega-3s
probably will be higher to regain something close
to a sane balance between these two groups of fats.
People with heart disease, inflammatory conditions,
a risk for dementia or depression also might need
higher doses of DHA than happy, disease-free folks.
Pregnancy and breast-feeding can deplete DHA stores
in the mother by up to 50%, so pregnant or lactating
women need at least 300 milligrams of DHA a day from
fish, fortified foods or supplements. In all other cases,
200 milligrams of DHA a day is a good starting point.

What About Supplements?

If you can't get at least 200 milligrams of DHA each
day from seafood or fortified foods (pregnant and
breast-feeding women need 300 milligrams), then

consider taking a supplement. Fish oil supplements are fine, but make sure to check the label. You want a supplement that spells out exactly how much DHA you are getting, not one that just lists the amount of fish oil. Some people complain of a few nasty side effects from fish oil capsules, such as burping or heartburn. Supplements of algae-based DHA also are available and are less likely to cause the fishy burping, especially when taken with meals or a glass of warm milk or orange juice.

When taking a supplement, always remember that just because some is good doesn't mean more is better. Omega-3s are blood thinners, so taking too much (such as more than 3 grams a day) could cause excessive bleeding. They should be taken only with a physician's approval if you are on blood-thinners, such as warfarin (coumadin) and other medications; aspirin; or high doses of vitamin E. Omega-3s also can lower blood pressure, so your doctor might want to lower the dosage on any blood pressure medications if you are taking DHA or other omega-3s. To be on the safe side, discuss any supplement, including fish oils or DHA, with your physician.

A Partial List of DHA Supplements

- Life Fitness—
  Life's DHA Prenatal
  Multivitamin & DHA

- Deva Omega-3 DHA

- Citracal® Prenatal
  + DHA

- Vitafol®-OB
  + DHA

- Spectrum Prenatal
  DHA

- Spectrum Children's
  DHA Chewable

- Spectrum Flax Oil with
  DHA

- Udo's DHA Oil Blend™

- Expecta™ LIPIL®

- NuTru O-Mega-Zen3®

- Pharmelle Natelle®
  Plus with DHA

- Spring Valley Plant-Pure
  Omega-3 DHA 200mg
  or 450mg

- Barleans Total Omega
  Vegan Swirl

- Walgreens-Pharmacist's
  Support Prenatal + DHA

- Pharmelle Natelle® Plus
  with DHA

How Much, of What and When?

DHA is a key factor in the diet of happy, fit people. You need at least 200 milligrams from fatty fish, foods fortified with DHA, or supplements. And you need to get that amount most days of the week. No ifs, ands or buts. Just do it!

SECRET 7:
GET SMART WITH SUPPLEMENTS

The Promise

**In one month of increasing
your intake of one or more
of these nutrients, you will:**

- think more clearly, more quickly
  and more creatively
- remember more
- notice an improvement in mood

In one year, you will:

- notice a more even, consistent good mood
- find that you are less likely to forget where you put
  your keys, cell phone and children
- feel less stressed
- sleep better
- note continued improvements in your mental clarity,
  problem-solving skills and reaction times

Ten years from now, you will:

- be at a lower risk for developing memory loss, dementia
  or even Alzheimer's disease
- continue to be happier and less stressed

A day without my supplements is a day destined for some unknown health disaster; I just don't feel completely safe without them! I make my family take them, too. Not too long ago, my daughter's friend told her mom, "If parents discipline their kids because they care, then Lauren's mom [that's me] must really love her, because she makes her take those nasty vitamins every day!"

Do I really need to take supplements to feel and think my best? Researchers at Tufts University might answer that question by saying nope, not if you eat really, really well (which I try to do). "Food is a complex package of vitamins, minerals, fiber and thousands of phytonutrients that are essential to health. With rare exceptions, there just isn't the evidence to support supplements over food in optimizing health or preventing disease," says Alice H. Lichtenstein, D.Sc., lead researcher on the Tufts commentary.

Jeffrey Blumberg, Ph.D., also at Tufts' Friedman School, agrees that food comes first: "That's why they are called *supplements*, not *substitutes*." But, he adds, there is plenty of evidence that supplements can fill in nutritional gaps in not-so-perfect diets—and maybe even lower risks for certain mood and mind conditions, such as depression and dementia. Besides, most nutrients are just as well absorbed from supplements as from foods, and some are even better taken in pill form!

For one thing, most people don't eat as well as they should and are marginally nourished in vitamins or minerals critical to their mood, minds and energy levels. Case in point: many women still fall far short of optimal levels for folic acid although even white bread and Pop Tarts are fortified with this B vitamin. Then there are studies that show people who supplement suffer less from a host of ills—ranging from premenstrual syndrome (PMS) to depression—compared to nonsupplementers. "It is self-evident that the immediate solution to this huge problem is for people to both improve their diets and also take dietary supplements to fill in the many large gaps between their current intake and the recommended amounts," concludes Dr. Blumberg.

It doesn't get any easier than taking a pill. With no side effects and some potentially amazing results, I don't understand why everyone doesn't take at least a multiple vitamin and mineral supplement. That's exactly what I told Chris, a dear friend and mother of two teenage boys.

For years, Chris dealt with dry skin patches on her face. She'd tried changing cleansers and bought expensive moisturizers, but no matter what she did, the dry skin wouldn't go away.

"Then, my mom came to visit. We always give her our master bedroom because the bathroom is more convenient for her. I forgot to get my proper cleansers and moisturizers from my bathroom, and, not wanting to wake my mother at 11:00 p.m. to rummage for my stuff in my bathroom I used any old soap in the boys' bathroom, and had to skip my usual moisturizing routine, knowing full well that my crazy skin would go nuts. Except that it didn't. No dry patches. No extra products, and my skin is smooth. The only difference in my routine that I could figure out was that I had taken Elizabeth's advice and just started taking a multiple. After three weeks, my skin issue is no longer an issue!"

Chris's story is one of many that have over the years convinced me to continue taking supplements. Yet faced with a wall of pills, powders and potions, it's a bit daunting trying to choose the right ones. Here's the lowdown on which supplements really might help improve your disposition and keep track of where you put your keys today and your memories tomorrow. Some might even be a help when dieting.

The Natural High

The right supplements taken in the right amounts can fill in the nutritional gaps on the days when you don't eat perfectly, and provide a helping hand when the body fails to make enough of some mood-boosting chemicals.

One Pill a Day

Most of your dietary woes are soothed if every day you eat at least eight servings of fresh fruits and vegetables, six servings of whole grains, three glasses of calcium-rich milk or soy milk, and two servings of extra-lean chicken, fish or legumes. Sounds reasonable, but there's a catch—finding anyone who does that is about as likely as trying to find someone who can walk on water.

The irony is most of us think we're eating pretty well. A Gallup poll conducted by the American Dietetic Association found that 90% of women surveyed said their diets were healthful. Most of them are delusional, since every national nutrition survey dating from the 1960s to the present repeatedly and consistently finds that most Americans don't come close to adequate, let alone optimal. Only one in every 100 people meet even minimum standards of the proverbial "balanced diet."

Even if you ate perfectly, no diet can realistically provide optimal amounts of certain nutrients. Take, for example,

- **Vitamin E.** You need at least 100 IU of this vitamin daily to cut the risk for memory loss and possibly Alzheimer's. Are you willing to eat 8 cups of almonds, ¾ cup safflower oil or 62 cups of fresh spinach every day to meet this need?
- **Calcium.** This mineral might help soothe the grumps in women seized with PMS. In fact, as

calcium intake goes up, so does mood for these women. The latest calcium recommendation to curb that bad mood is 1,000 to 1,200 milligrams daily, which is easy enough if you drink four glasses of milk or soy milk daily. For those people who shun milk, meeting this quota means consuming 6 ounces of tofu, a can of salmon with the bones, and 2 cups of black bean soup every day.

- **Folic acid.** This B vitamin is critical to mood and memory, but even though white flour and all the junk food made from it are now fortified with folic acid, intakes still fall short for a huge section of the population. You need at least two servings every day of foods rich in folate, like greens. But when researchers at the University of California, Berkeley investigated women's intake of dark green leafies, they found almost 9 out of every 10 women failed to include even one serving on any one of four days!

- **Vitamin D.** Frankly, I don't know where anyone gets enough of this vitamin, since even drinking four glasses of fortified milk or soy milk daily won't meet current needs for most people, and the amount of time you must spend in direct overhead sun without sunscreen is totally unrealistic, especially in the winter. Yet not getting enough of this vitamin is a big mistake if you battle mood, memory or possibly even weight issues.

Happy, fit people know that to improve their moods, sharpen their minds, lift energy and fill in nutritional gaps while dieting, it's a smart idea to take a moderate-dose, balanced multivitamin and mineral supplement. There is even evidence that a moderate-dose multi can lessen depression, improve mood, reduce stress and anxiety and soothe troubled emotions.

This makes sense since most vitamins and minerals are assembly-line workers in the brain. For example, the B vitamins convert glucose into energy for the brain and also help build some of the nerve chemicals that then tell you to cry at a sad place in a book or laugh at the right spot in a movie. Vitamin D protects nerves in the brain from degenerating. Vitamin E protects brain cell membranes from aging. Iron ensures your brain gets enough oxygen. Iodine ensures normal brain metabolism. The list goes on and on.

Supplements versus Food

Sure, you still need to eat right, but nutrition and supplements are not an either-or issue. The two enhance each together, not cancel each other out. You don't always get optimal amounts of all the vitamins and minerals from food, just as pills don't contain everything that food has to offer.

For one thing, supplements can replace the vitamins and minerals, but they will never supply the thousands of other health-enhancing phytonutrients obtained from real foods. Second, while a well-chosen supplement can improve some of the nutritional shortcomings of a good diet, it can't compensate for bad eating habits. You know deep down in your heart that you can't live on French fries and hamburgers, then take a vitamin E supplement and think you're doing fine. So eat right, but also take a multi as a good safety net for those days when you eat well, but not well enough.

What should you look for in a multi?

- Select a broad-range multiple vitamin and mineral supplement. Choose one that contains vitamins A, D, E and K, all of the B vitamins (vitamins B_1, B_2, B_6, B_{12}, niacin and folic acid), and the trace minerals (chromium, copper, iron, manganese, selenium and zinc).

- Ignore chloride, pantothenic acid, biotin, potassium, choline and phosphorus since the diet either already supplies optimal levels of these compounds or supplements contain too little to be useful. Also ignore nickel, iodine, vanadium and tin, since it's not clear whether they're essential for people.

- Read the column titled "Daily Value" on the back label. Look for a multiple that provides approximately 100%, but no more than 300% of the Daily Value for all nutrients provided. You want a "balanced" supplement, not one that supplies 2% of one nutrient, 50% of another, and 600% of another.

- Supplement your multi. All one-pill-a-day multiples are short on calcium and magnesium, so consider taking a calcium-magnesium supplement if you consume less than three glasses of milk and several servings of magnesium-rich soybeans, wheat germ and dark green leafy vegetables each day. Look for one that supplies these two minerals in a two to one ratio, such as 500 milligrams of calcium to 250 milligrams of magnesium.

The Top Five Most Frequently Asked Questions About Supplements

1. How can I cut down on cost without sacrificing quality?
Avoid the "extra" ingredients, such as lipoic acid, enzymes, primrose oil or inositol, to name only a few. These extras add cost, not value, since they are either worthless or supplied in amounts too low to be of use. Also, avoid the "natural" products; they're costly and usually provide no added benefit over other supplements. Then purchase bigger or "economy size" bottles when the unit price saves you money, and use the supplements before the expiration date.

2. Are time-release vitamins and chelated minerals better than regular supplements? No. These products are more show than substance. Most time-release supplements dissolve too slowly to be completely absorbed. Taking your multiple in divided doses throughout the day is a better, and less expensive, alternative. There is no convincing evidence that chelated or colloidal minerals are any better absorbed or used by the body than other minerals.

3. When's the best time of day to take a supplement? The time of day is not as important as what you take them with. Most nutrients are best absorbed when taken with meals and taken in divided doses throughout the day. Take a multiple with iron at a different meal than your calcium supplement, since these two minerals compete for absorption.

4. What do the letters USP mean on a supplement label? United States Pharmacopeia or USP is a nongovernmental standard-setting body. This seal of quality means the supplement should dissolve within the digestive tract, is made from pure ingredients and contains the amount of nutrients listed on the label.

5. Can I trust the claims on the label? Usually not. Claims that a product is "complete," "balanced," "high potency" or "specially formulated," contains "extra antioxidants" or is a "multivitamin or multimineral" have little to do with the real formulations. Claims that a supplement will cure, treat or even prevent any health condition are more hype than fact.

Antioxidants for an Antiaging Brain

Your body "rusts" when exposed to little oxygen fragments called free radicals or oxidants. Our bodies and brains are exposed to these troublemakers when we breathe air pollution and tobacco smoke, eat fatty foods and are exposed to pesticides. Even if you lived in a pristine world, your body still would be making free radicals during normal metabolic processes. (See Chapter 5 for more about antioxidants and free radicals.)

Luckily, your body has an anti-free radical arsenal, called antioxidants. These are the house-keepers that sweep up oxidants and flush them out of the body. Antioxidants defend cells from aging and protect tiny blood vessels that transport nutrients to brain cells, keeping them elastic and free of "debris." Since 20% of the heart's output goes to the brain, all of these benefits mean improved blood flow and better thinking.

The trick is to maintain an antioxidant arsenal equal to or better than the onslaught of free radicals. As we get older, oxidative damage to tissues, including the brain, intensifies, so that a 30-year-old person needs more antioxidants than a teenager, and the required dose increases even more with every passing decade. If you want to protect your brain, you must build a huge antioxidant arsenal, then replenish it daily.

And it works. People who feast on antioxidant-rich foods and supplements throughout the day also have the highest blood and tissue levels of these do-gooders and the lowest risk for developing dementia, depression or even Alzheimer's disease. They live the longest, they think the clearest and they are the happiest. Even their sex lives improve!

From Vitamins to Phytonutrients

You probably already know that vitamins C and E and other nutrients like selenium are big-time antioxidants that reduce the risk for memory loss. They work much better as a team than supplied alone.

There are literally thousands of compounds in real foods, like herbs, whole grains, legumes, and colorful fruits and vegetables, called phytonutrients. They aren't vitamins or minerals. Instead, they are compounds with potent antioxidant abilities, especially when supplied as teams. There are the flavonoids in citrus, anthocyanins in red cabbage and cherries, lycopene in tomatoes and watermelon, lutein in spinach, sulforaphane in broccoli, ellagic acid in berries and sulfur compounds in garlic, to name only a few.

Not only do these phytonutrients protect the brain and body from free radical damage, but they also tickle the genetic code within all your body's cells, turning on the natural production of your body's own antioxidants, which then protect your brain 24/7 from damage. In other words, taking a vitamin C pill is great, but short-lived, while getting enough of the right mix of phytonutrients means your brain is protected around the clock.

What's this got to do with supplements?

- *First,* if you don't load the menu every day with real or super mood foods, it's a good idea to

take an antioxidant supplement that contains
vitamin C and vitamin E. Aim for at least
250 milligrams of vitamin C and at least 100 IU
of vitamin E. Take it in divided doses if you
can, since nutrients are best absorbed and
best used in the body when they are supplied
in small, frequent doses.

- *Second,* skip supplements that pride themselves on supplying a smattering of a few
phytonutrients, like lutein or lycopene. They
are a scam. No one even knows how much of
each phytochemical we need or how they work
in tandem.

- *Third,* there are a few new supplements on the
market that actually do work, such as Protandim.
They aren't antioxidants themselves, but they
contain a mix of phytonutrients that turn on
your body's production of its own antioxidants.
They work to reduce free radicals and potentially
protect your brain. Supplements like Protandim
are a whole new approach to cellular health.
They naturally increase your body's production
of two antioxidant enzymes that aid in eliminating free radicals in your cells, helping to decrease
cellular damage and promote healthy aging and
immune function.

While all the 40+ nutrients are critical to your happiness quotient, a few vitamins, minerals and other

compounds are superheroes in the fight against depression, fatigue, memory loss, and more. Here's the short list on the ones most important to your mood.

B Good to Yourself

If you feel down in the dumps, too pooped to play or can't remember your own name, then it just might be that you aren't getting enough of the B vitamins.

That's what Darlene, a teacher in Albuquerque, learned after suffering debilitating exhaustion and depression. She brushed it off—and the 25-pound weight gain that accompanied it—as the start of premenopause. Her physician put her on a stew of medications, from antidepressants to thyroid hormones. "Sure, the drugs helped improve my mood," she says, "but I wanted to get to the root of the problem, so I found a doctor who was willing to work with me on alternative approaches."

As Darlene slowly weaned herself off the antidepressants, she replaced them with supplements of B vitamins, along with omega-3 fats and several other nutrients known to affect mood (such as calcium, magnesium, vitamin D, zinc and vitamin E). "The transition was seamless. I felt energized, positive, eager to get up in the morning, yet was finally off all medications!" What's more, the weight dropped off without her even trying.

The Bs are everywhere in the brain. Some B vitamins, especially vitamins B_1, B_2, and pantothenic acid, help release energy to brain cells so you can think straight. Some Bs, like vitamin B_6 and folic acid, are star attractions in making nerve chemicals that keep you happy (like serotonin). Other Bs, like vitamin B_{12}, build the insulation sheath around brain cells that allow messages to travel lickety-split from one cell to another. Include enough of these in your diet and you think fast, feel good and have lots of energy.

Folic Acid: Nature's Blues Buster

As many as one in every three Americans doesn't get enough folic acid, the B vitamin important in making sure your brain cells multiply correctly, in boosting levels of the brain-building omega-3 fat DHA and in ensuring your brain makes enough of the feel-good chemicals serotonin and SAM-e (more on this later in this chapter). Low intake of this B vitamin alone increases the risk for being depressed by up to 67%.

People who are serious about getting enough folic acid are the ones most likely to be happy, mentally sharp and at low risk for dementia, depression and Alzheimer's. If they are depressed, increasing their folic acid speeds recovery. Better yet, folic acid is better absorbed from supplements than from food, so you can rest assured you are getting enough when you take it in pill form.

A word of caution: large doses of supplemental folic acid can mask a vitamin B_{12} deficiency, so to be on the safe side, take extra B_{12} if you are supplementing daily with more than 400 micrograms of folic acid.

Vitamin B_6: The Good Mood Vitamin

More than one in four people with depression are deficient in vitamin B_6. Boosting intake, either from food or supplements, often is all it takes to see an improvement in their moods. Vitamin B_6 (along with vitamin B_{12}) combined with antidepressant medications even provides a better mood boost than medications alone.

B_6 also seems to help people cope better with stress. For example, women with premenstrual syndrome (PMS) often feel stressed out and crabby before their periods. Or it might be connected to the form of birth control they choose. Birth control pills partially block vitamin B_6 activity in the body, so nerve cells are unable to manufacture adequate amounts of serotonin.

Take a supplement that contains 5 milligrams (but no more than 150 milligrams) of vitamin B_6 if you aren't vigilant in getting several B_6-rich foods into your daily diet, such as chicken breast, bananas, fish or whole grains.

Vitamin B$_{12}$: Maximum Brain Support

The mind shuts down without vitamin B$_{12}$. It might even start shrinking! You need this B vitamin to ensure your brain cells can send messages back and forth quickly, so you have no trouble putting two words together, remembering a friend's name or staying quick-witted. It's no wonder that studies, like one from the University of Oxford, repeatedly find that you lose your ability to think, remember and react in direct proportion to your B$_{12}$ levels. Even happy people tend to tumble into depression when B$_{12}$ levels are low. Studies show that people with markers for low vitamin B$_{12}$ status have a more rapid drop-off in mental function at younger ages compared to people with optimal vitamin B$_{12}$ status. In fact, many researchers speculate that doubling a person's vitamin B$_{12}$ levels by taking supplements could slow cognitive decline by one-third or more.

Even people who are tested for vitamin B$_{12}$ and are found to be in the low-normal range could be deficient, according to a study from the University of Oxford. Tamara knows firsthand how powerful an influence vitamin B$_{12}$ has on mood. She had battled serious depression for five years despite taking a variety of antidepressant medications. In desperation and at the age of 42 years, she turned to her doctors one more time for help. Routine blood tests had shown she wasn't anemic or even low in B$_{12}$, but her doctor decided to put her on supplemental vitamin B_{12} and folic acid anyway. Within weeks, her depression completely vanished. A year later, she was still blues-free. "I've not had a miserable day since," she adds.

Many studies also find that people living in nursing homes because of memory loss often improve beyond anyone's wildest dreams when they are given high doses of vitamin B_{12}.

The older you are, the more vitamin B_{12} you need, with young people needing as little as 2 micrograms a day, while anyone over the age of 50 years needs at least 25 micrograms, maybe more. It would be difficult to get that much from diet alone, and besides, vitamin B_{12} is another nutrient better absorbed from supplements than from foods. You might even need to take shots instead of pills.

Vitamin B_{12} requires a substance in the stomach, called Intrinsic Factor, for absorption. Ample stomach acid is needed to trigger intrinsic factor, but acid often decreases as a person ages and definitely decreases when people take antacids or other medications for heartburn. Consequently, risk for vitamin B_{12} deficiency increases steadily as some people get older. Increased supplemental intake of this vitamin can offset this reduced absorption in many cases, but some people might require vitamin B_{12} shots, especially if they are on heartburn medications or have low stomach acid.

Gimme a D!

Vitamin D is no longer just for strong bones. In fact, it might be useful for a whole host of ills, from diabetes, multiple sclerosis, cancer and heart disease to boosting your immune system, curing chronic muscle pain and fibromyalgia and preventing depression, anxiety and even memory loss. There are even suspicions that a deficiency increases the risk for obesity. What's more, you possibly need a whole lot more than you think. Happy, fit people place this vitamin at the top of their to-do list.

Up until recently, vitamin D's only known job was to help prevent bone loss associated with diseases like osteoporosis and rickets. That's because vitamin D is critical for the absorption of calcium and also ensuring the mineral gets deposited into bones. If you're low on vitamin D, it's a given you'll only absorb about 10% of the calcium you consume, which is a surefire way to end up with osteoporosis later in life, even if you take lots of calcium. Getting enough vitamin D and calcium can significantly improve a woman's chances of avoiding osteoporosis.

While we used to think only bones were sensitive to vitamin D, experts are finding that almost every tissue in the body has receptors for vitamin D, suggesting that it works its magic everywhere in the body.

We now know that vitamin D aids in the prevention and/or treatment of gum disease, diabetes, insulin resistance, arthritis, multiple sclerosis, hypertension and certain cancers, including colon, breast, pancreas and prostate cancers. Vitamin D also reduces the incidence of falls by up to 60% in seniors. A few very recent studies even suggest that vitamin D is critical for brain function in general, helping to boost not just mood, but also memory, reaction times and thinking.

In addition, we know that a deficiency of this vitamin is typically found in people who have risk factors for obesity, such as heart disease, diabetes and high blood pressure. It also is clear that overweight people are prime candidates for a vitamin D deficiency.

Happy, fit people also might get their mood boost from this vitamin. People prone to the blues have low levels of vitamin D, while happy people's vitamin D levels are much higher. Even healthy, relatively happy people report a mood boost when they add extra vitamin D to their diets. The research is strongest for people battling seasonal affective disorder, or SAD, whose mood worsens as the seasons progress from fall through winter. For years, the only known cause was thought to be lack of sunlight. But it might be vitamin D these people lack.

Vitamin D really isn't a vitamin at all. It's a hormone. You don't need to get it from your diet, since your body can make vitamin D if it's exposed to sunlight long enough. When it comes to SAD, it might not be the lack of sunlight that causes the winter blues, but rather the lack of sunlight means the body can't make enough vitamin D, which otherwise would have sparked a perkier mood through the winter months.

That's what the research shows. Deficiencies of vitamin D escalate from 38% to 60% from fall to spring in people who battle SAD. Give them extra doses of vitamin D, and voilà! Their mood improves and anxiety drops. Although not yet studied, winter depression typically goes hand in hand with weight gain. Sidestep the blues and you might have a better chance of fitting into a swimsuit by spring.

A Cure for Muscle Aches?

Depression and muscle aches also might be a sign you are low in this vitamin. In fact, the depression, as well as the muscle and bone aches in a vitamin D deficiency, mimic the symptoms of fibromyalgia. Boost intake of this vitamin and the pain vanishes, while mood improves. Researchers suspect that up to 90% of unexplained chronic muscle pain could result from poor vitamin D status.

D-ficient?

Your body can make vitamin D, so why worry about whether you're getting enough? Maybe because most Americans are deficient! In fact, more than 60% of Americans are woefully low in this vitamin. Nearly half of all people who take a supplement and think they are fine are actually deficient. That's because four very important factors affect how well and how much vitamin D we make and, therefore, whether we are at risk for deficiency.

1. Age: Our bodies make vitamin D when skin is exposed to UVB sunlight. However, a person's ability to manufacture vitamin D decreases with each passing decade, so by the time people enter their senior years, their bodies make as little as 20% of the vitamin D they made in childhood. In short, the older they are, the greater the risk for deficiency.

2. Location: People living north of the latitude running generally through Los Angeles and Atlanta typically are sun deprived and, consequently, low in vitamin D, especially during fall and winter. A recent study from the University of Georgia found that 75% of young girls had low blood levels for vitamin D, potentially placing them at risk for disease. If that many young girls living in sunny climates are low, it's no wonder researchers suspect that everyone living in the north is low in vitamin D.

3. Skin Color: Melanin is the pigment that gives skin its color. Greater amounts of melanin result in darker skin. The high melanin content in darker skin reduces the skin's ability to produce vitamin D from sunlight, which explains why African-Americans with a high level of melanin in their skin are 10 times more likely to be vitamin D deficient compared to fair-skinned people. Some studies suggest that older adults, especially women, in these groups are at even higher risk of vitamin D deficiency.

4. Sunscreen: Sunscreen blocks harmful UVB rays that cause skin cancer. That's a good thing. But sunscreen also blocks the skin's ability to make vitamin D. Even a sunscreen with an SPF of 8 blocks vitamin D by 97.5%. So people who lavishly use sunscreen can develop a deficiency, even if they are out in the sun all day.

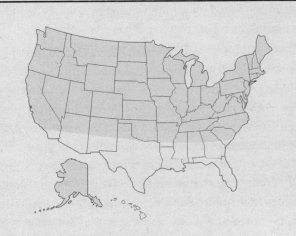

Who Doesn't Get Enough?

If you live anywhere above an imaginary line drawn between Los Angeles, California, and Atlanta, Georgia, you probably are not getting enough sunlight during the fall, winter and even spring months to ensure optimal vitamin D intake.

How Much Do You Need?

Up until recently, vitamin D was considered one of the vitamins that could be toxic, so safe intake limits were set very low, or about 200 IU to 600 IU a day, depending on age. But all the studies showing vitamin D lowers risk for everything from muscle pain to depression have used amounts far in excess of what people typically consume and, in many cases, much more than the current daily recommendations. As a result, many experts are calling for a change in the recommendations, which were set back in 1997 and are considered outdated and too restrictive.

According to researchers at Harvard, a supplement containing 1,000 IU a day would be helpful to the vast majority of Americans. The likelihood of toxicity at this dose is nonexistent. Hey, fair-skinned people's bodies can manufacture 15,000 IU or more in as little as 30 minutes of unprotected sunbathing in the middle of July, so 1,000 IU is a pretty safe dose to consider! Of course, you should always consult your physician before taking any supplement, but for people living in the north or anyone over the age of 50, some type of vitamin D supplement is well worth pondering.

As with any nutrient, just because some is good doesn't mean more is better. Vitamin D is a fat-soluble vitamin, which means the body doesn't get rid of it when it is in excess, but rather stores it for future use. Build up too high a store and you could end up with kidney stones or even start stockpiling calcium in your heart or arteries, places that shouldn't be hardened with bone minerals!

You can play on the safe side and have your level of this vitamin measured next time you are going in for a blood draw anyway. Ask to be tested for 25-hydroxy Vitamin D. A value below 20 nanograms is low, 20 to 30 nanograms is borderline and 30 to 50 nanograms is optimal. Have the test in November, because if you are low then, it is a sure thing you'll be full-blown deficient by spring.

Light, Food and Supplements

Where are you going to get your D? You have three choices: 1. spend time in the direct sun, 2. eat lots of foods rich in this vitamin and 3. take a supplement. The first option is near impossible. Either you live south of Los Angeles and Atlanta and have not heeded the warnings to use sunscreen to prevent skin cancer, or you are at risk for a vitamin D deficiency. The second option also is difficult, since so few foods naturally contain much vitamin D and fortified foods are limited to no more than 100 IU per serving. That means you must drink 10 glasses of milk a day to get the latest recommended intake of 1,000 IU a day. Not likely.

That leaves supplements. If you live in hot, sunny climates and drink some milk or soy milk, then aim for 400 IU from supplements to fill in the gaps. For everyone else, talk to your physician about taking a supplement of 1000 IU a day.

Iron Up, Ladies

If you are a woman who feels down in the dumps or downright depressed much of the time, or if your energy level has taken a nosedive, rather than reach for another cup of coffee to get yourself through the day, try a little iron therapy.

Iron deficiency is the number one most prevalent nutrient deficiency, with estimates as high as 50% of women of childbearing age to 80% of active women being iron deficient. It's almost a given if you are between the ages of 13 to 50, have been pregnant in the past two years, consume less than 2,000 calories daily, menstruate heavily or exercise frequently and vigorously that your iron levels are low. In contrast, seldom do men or postmenopausal women need to worry about iron; they should consider supplements only if blood tests show they are deficient, and even then only with physician monitoring.

Give Me Oxygen, or Give Me Death!

What's the big deal with iron? This little trace mineral is the key oxygen carrier in the blood. Without enough iron, the tissues literally suffocate for oxygen and the signs of deficiency reflect this: you are fatigued, feel sluggish, can't concentrate and are likely to come down with every cold and flu bug that passes by. You also are more prone to depression, postpartum depression, stress, anxiety, irritability, lethargy and memory loss. If you are a student, you have trouble retaining information, doing well on tests or even staying awake during class. If you exercise, you might notice that you can't recover as quickly from an exercise session, your muscle strength is declining and you tire easily.

Those symptoms might sound like anemia, but it's not likely you are anemic. Anemia is the final stage of iron deficiency. For months, years, even decades, you can be iron deficient and never progress to anemia. In fact, only about 8% of women actually become anemic, while anywhere between 20% and 80% of women are iron deficient. Long before the onset of anemia, tissue iron reserves are drained.

Request the Right Test

Your doctor typically only checks for anemia, drawing blood for hemoglobin and hematocrit tests. These tests pick up full-blown anemia, while more subtle iron deficiency goes unnoticed. That's why if you suspect iron deficiency, you should request a more sensitive test called the "serum ferritin" test. And don't be satisfied with a diagnosis of "you're fine." Ask for the value. A value of less than 20 mcg/l means you are iron deficient.

It happened to me when I was pregnant with my first child. I was an avid runner, averaging 40 or more miles a week, but now I could hardly make it up the short flight of stairs to my office in San Diego. When I complained to my doctor, he shrugged it off. "Of course you are tired, you're pregnant. Your blood-work looks fine, just take it a little easier." I knew how I felt wasn't normal, so I ordered my own serum ferritin test. Instead of the optimal value of 20 or higher, my value was a measly 4 micrograms. When I returned to my doctor's office and showed him the results, his attitude changed. "Well, I'll be. You are iron deficient." He put me on prescription iron supplements and within two weeks I was bounding up the stairs to my office again.

That experience convinced me how subtle, yet devastating, low iron can be. I knew how to eat right, yet even I was deficient. How many more women who weren't trained to be as nutrition savvy as me were slugging it through the day, getting by with coffee and colas to stay awake, when really what they needed was a good kick in their iron intake? From then on, I asked every teenage girl and woman who came to me complaining of muddled thinking or feeling drained of energy to go back to their doctors and demand a serum ferritin test. You know what? Every single one of them that took the test found they were iron deficient.

Ironclad Rules

The best plan to avoid iron deficiency is prevention, but women must get much more aggressive about their iron intakes, since currently most of us average only about half our daily needs. Premenopausal women should consume several iron-rich foods daily, including extra-lean meat, fish, poultry and super mood foods like cooked dried beans and peas, dried apricots, dark green leafy vegetables and whole grains. They also should

1. Consume a vitamin C—rich food with every meal. Try orange juice, a tossed salad, broccoli or most fruits. Vitamin C dramatically improves the absorption of iron and counteracts some of the inhibitors in foods, such as phytates in whole grains and tannins in tea and coffee.

2. Emphasize the best iron. There are two types of dietary iron: the iron in meat, called heme iron, and the iron in plants, called nonheme iron. Heme iron is really well absorbed; about 30% of it makes it into the bloodstream, compared to only 2% to 7% of nonheme iron. Consuming small amounts of heme iron in red meat, such as extra-lean beef, with large amounts of nonheme iron, such as chili beans, increases the absorption of nonheme iron. Pork in a vegetable stir-fry and spaghetti with meatballs are other examples.

3. Cook in a cast iron skillet. The iron leaches out of the pot into the food, raising the iron content several hundred-fold, especially with acid foods, like tomato and spaghetti sauce.

4. Select iron-fortified foods. Choose foods with extra iron, such as ready-to-eat cereals or fortified oatmeal.

5. Drink tea and coffee between meals. Compounds called tannins in these beverages, whether they are caffeinated or decaffeinated or herb, green or black teas, block iron absorption by up to 80% when drunk with a meal.

6. Take iron supplements on an empty stomach to improve absorption. The best-absorbed forms are the "ferrous" forms, such as ferrous fumarate or ferrous sulfate.

A moderate-dose iron supplement should be considered when food intake falls below 2,500 calories and serum ferritin levels fall below 20mcg/l. How much? Premenopausal women need 18 milligrams of iron daily, while pregnant women need at least 27 milligrams. (Postmenopausal women and men need as little as 8 to 10 milligrams from food.) Women who are vegetarians, who menstruate heavily or who are on the IUD for birth control might need even higher amounts, up to 25 milligrams.

Unless prescribed by a physician, postmenopausal women should not take supplemental iron or should limit intake to no more than 10 milligrams. Severe iron deficiency may require a higher-dose prescription supplement. Supplements are just as effective as food in raising iron levels in the body, but you are best doing both—eating lots of iron-rich foods and taking a moderate-dose multiple that contains iron.

Iron is one of the few nutrients that can easily be assessed by a simple blood test. Feeling "not up to par" might not be all in your head, so don't take it lying down!

The Antistress Mineral

Magnesium gets no respect. Other nutrients, like calcium, folic acid or iron, are in the news all the time, and even vitamin D has been getting some press of late. But you never hear about magnesium. Big mistake.

This mineral helps in more than 300 processes in the body. In fact, every cell in your body needs this mineral. That might explain why it helps lower the risk for diabetes, heart disease, high blood pressure, osteoporosis and much more. Yet three out of four Americans don't get enough.

Why Magnesium?

When it comes to mood, magnesium is a major player. Stress triggers the release of stress hormones that drain magnesium from the body. In turn, low magnesium levels raise stress hormones, escalating the stress response. Studies on animals show that low magnesium intake increases sensitivity to noise and crowding and escalates stress-induced diseases, such as ulcers, while animals fed magnesium-rich diets cope better and are at lower risk for disease. Studies on people under pressure at work to meet ridiculously tight deadlines cope far better when their diets are rich in magnesium but are more likely to freak out if they aren't.

Women who get crabby, depressed and downright difficult to live with the 10 to 14 days before their periods also need more magnesium. Magnesium levels drop during the last two weeks of the menstrual cycle, which might contribute to PMS symptoms, such as water retention, cramping, headaches and an oversensitive nervous system (feeling crabby, irritable and edgy?). Increasing intake of magnesium helps curb these symptoms—even to recommended levels is enough to see improvement in symptoms for some women.

How Much Do You Need?

You need about 320 to 500 milligrams of this feel-good nutrient every day. That doesn't sound like much until you realize that most of the magnesium gold mines in the diet are foods many people don't typically include in generous amounts, such as avocados, oysters, bananas and the super mood foods wheat germ, whole grains, cooked dried beans and peas and dark green leafy vegetables.

If you choose to supplement, look for the best absorbed forms, such as magnesium oxide, citrate or hydroxide. But don't go overboard on this mineral! It is the active ingredient in Milk of Magnesia, which means that too much can loosen more than your muscles, leaving you in the bathroom rather than at the party.

Sammy Baby

For anyone battling depression, just getting up in the morning can be an overwhelming chore. The thought that there could be a natural solution with no side effects and that it's as easy as taking a pill is almost too good to be true. But it is. Thirty years of studies show that SAM-e—the user-friendly name for S-adenosylmethionine—is as effective, and maybe even more effective, than some antidepressant medications in relieving the symptoms of depression.

SAM-e (pronounced "sammy") isn't a hormone, herb, vitamin or nutrient. It's made naturally in the body from an amino acid called methionine, which you get from protein-rich foods, along with the assembly-line workers folic acid and vitamin B_{12}.

Sometimes the body doesn't make enough. This can cause all kinds of problems, since SAM-e acts as the "on" switch for a wide variety of processes.

It helps make new cells and repair damaged ones, aids immunity, builds cartilage in joints, helps form the genetic code within cells, makes nerve chemicals like serotonin and dopamine and regulates moods and emotions. This translates into happier moods, quicker thinking, reduced arthritis pain and possibly fewer symptoms of fibromyalgia.

It is with mood that SAM-e works its best magic. Low SAM-e levels are seen in people who are depressed. Raise those levels by supplementing with SAM-e and despair, anxiety and irritability improve, if not vanish.

Numerous studies show that SAM-e works when all else fails. One study found that 400 milligrams a day of SAM-e was even more effective at eliminating depression than mood-altering medications. This supplement bests antidepressant drugs because it starts working within a few days to two weeks, while prescription drugs take much longer. SAM-e also appears to have few, if any, side effects, other than the occasional rare case of indigestion.

SAM-e also might be a smart pill, helping you concentrate and think faster. In one study, a combination of nutrients, including folic acid, vitamin B_{12}, vitamin E and SAM-e, improved quick thinking by 10% in just three months and by 20% at the end of a six-month study. Preliminary evidence also suggests this little pill might help curb Alzheimer's risk.

Are there any downsides to SAM-e? Yes, but they are few:

- While up to 61% of depressed people get relief with this supplement, there is no evidence that it has any effect on mood in people who are already happy. It shouldn't be taken as a tonic unless you really are blue.
- SAM-e is off-limits for anyone with bipolar disorder, since it can escalate manic episodes.
- Other than the fact that SAM-e has been used safely in Europe for more than 30 years as an antidepressant, there are few long-term studies, so no one knows for sure whether there might be any serious health hazards from taking it for decades.
- It's expensive, and analyses have found that what is promised on the label is not always what is inside the jar. Some brands have little or no SAM-e in their products, others have too much. To make sure you are getting what you paid for, choose a major brand, like NatureMade, to ensure quality.

How Much Do You Need?

Always discuss with your physician whether SAM-e is right for you. If you get the go-ahead, it typically is recommended that you start with 200 to 400 milligrams a day and up the dosage by 200 milligrams if you don't see results within two weeks. Some studies have used up to 1,200 to 1,600 milligrams a day. Look for brands that list 1,4-Butanedisulfonate on the label. That's an ingredient in the patented formulation of SAM-e used in Europe. Also look for products that are enteric-coated, which ensures they remain intact through the stomach and don't dissolve until they get into the small intestine, where they are absorbed into the bloodstream.

Herbal Remedies for a Bad Mood

- **St. John's Wort:** Also called hypericum, this herb curbs symptoms of depression in about one in every two people battling mild depression, SAD and possibly even PMS. No optimal dose has been identified, but a suggested dose is 300 to 1,800 milligrams a day, taken in divided doses. Always discuss this herb with your physician before taking, since it can interfere with some medications, including oral contraceptives, warfarin (Coumadin) and Cyclosporin, and should not be taken with antidepressant drugs.

- **Kava Kava:** Fans swear this herb calms them down, is a painkiller and helps them think clearly. Kava lactones in kava kava tickle the processing centers for emotions and moods in the brain. But studies have produced mixed results. When kava kava does work, the effective dose appears to be somewhere around 100 milligrams of kava extract taken three times a day. Look for products standardized to contain at least 70% kava lactones (60 to 75 milligrams/capsule). Don't take this antianxiety herb with prescription medications, when driving or operating heavy equipment, with alcohol or if you are younger than 21 years old, pregnant or nursing.

- **Gingko:** This root possibly boosts memory and attention, improves circulation, and aids in the treatment of dementia, tinnitus and Alzheimer's disease. You need at least 120 milligrams a day, preferably in divided doses. Look for products standardized to 24% flavone glycosides and 6% terpene lactones. Gingko might upset your stomach, cause headaches or skin reactions, and it should not be taken by pregnant women, before surgery or in conjunction with blood-thinning medications, including aspirin. Always consult your physician if you are taking any prescription medications.

- **Ginseng:** Studies on animals show ginseng might aid the nerves and heart and help balance hormones, promote immunity and boost metabolism, improve thinking and memory and even slow aging. Benefits for people are unknown, but possibly include helping control blood sugar in diabetics. You need 0.5 to 2 grams of the dried root, or up to ½ teaspoon ginseng extract or tea taken up to twice daily. Many ginseng supplements contain less active ingredients than listed on the label or are contaminated with lead or pesticides, so stick with reputable brands that are standardized to 4% to 7% ginsenosides. Take for no longer than three months. Pregnant and breast-feeding women or anyone with high blood pressure should avoid ginseng. Diabetics should be monitored by a physician.

Happiness in a Pill

All of these supplements can help improve mood and are relatively safe when taken in the recommended doses. But don't get carried away. You can't cover your bases with a pill, so don't leave common sense and good nutrition waiting in the wings. You must eat really well and supplement responsibly if you want to feel, look, think and act younger than your age!

If you're hungry for more info on supplements, check out the National Institutes of Medicine Office of Dietary Supplements website at www.ods.od.nih.gov.

SECRET 8:
CHOOSE THE RIGHT THIRST QUENCHERS

The Promise

**In one week of making
this change, you will:**

- have more energy

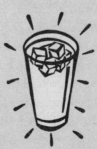

In one month, you will:

- drop up to 2 pounds
- notice an improvement in mood

In one year, you will:

- lose up to 26 pounds
- feel great
- have more energy

Sarah, a flight attendant from Chula Vista, California, stuck to her diet like glue. She had a bowl of cereal with nonfat milk and fruit in the morning. At lunch, she alternated between a turkey sandwich on whole wheat and a veggie wrap. At dinner, she paid close attention to just the right 3-ounce portion of meat with lots of vegetables. She exercised most days of the week and kept her snacks to a minimum. Yet she didn't lose a single pound. "It was so discouraging," she says. "After six weeks, I was no closer to my weight goal, so what was the point of even trying!" A glance at her diet showed little room for improvement. She wasn't snacking on the airline peanuts or finishing off her husband's French fries at restaurants. She passed my correct-portion size test and had cut out all sweets. Sarah was either lying about what she was eating and how much she was exercising, or she was defying the laws of physics.

Turns out she wasn't exactly lying, it just didn't occur to her that the few drinks she had with coworkers after a long flight could possibly do so much damage to her dieting efforts, let alone her mood. Repeated questioning finally uncovered that two or three times a week, Sarah had a couple of margaritas or Long Island Iced Teas. She also was partial to bottled green tea. What she didn't know was those thirst quenchers added 1,500 to 2,000 calories to her diet, which offset the 500 calories she had cut back each day. "I thought the tea was calorie-free—what a shock to find it had more calories than three cookies!" she groaned. The drinks while socializing and a bottle of tea every day was all it took to erase all the dieting efforts all week long! Like Sarah, it is easy to undo all of your best efforts to be healthy, fit and happy, not by what you load onto your plate, but by what you pour into your glass or chug out of a bottle.

Samantha was a doctoral student with me at Ohio State (in health education, no less!). I'll never forget the time she casually mentioned to me that she chugged two liters of cola every night while studying. My mouth dropped to my knees. That's 850 calories of sugar water. If she did that every day for a year, she'd have consumed 310,250 empty calories—the equivalent of 88 pounds of body fat!

A Cosmopolitan or apple martini during happy hour, a soft drink while watching TV or a bottle of vitamin water to quench thirst is such a natural accompaniment to visiting with friends or unwinding at the end of the day that we sometimes forget about the calories we are consuming. Big mistake. Ignoring calories in beverages often undermines our best efforts to be fit, happy and healthy.

The Natural High

Water is the most important nutrient in our diets. Second only to oxygen, it is hands-down, absolutely critical for life. Just make sure you get your water from no- or low-calorie options, so you nourish your body, mind and mood without packing on the pounds.

Liquid Calories

Not only are some drinks calorific, but those liquid calories are more fattening than calories in solid foods. They fly under our appetite-control radar, so they don't fill us up. The calories in a root beer or a mojito are calories added to our total day's intake, rather than replacing some of the calories in solid foods. It's as if the internal calorie counter in our brains that keeps track of incoming calories is blind to liquids. So when we have a soda, we eat just as much at the meal as we would if we drank water. But the soda added 250 calories on top of the meal, while the water was calorie free.

This explains why study after study shows that the more bottled sugar water people drink in the form of soft drinks, bottled coffee drinks or teas, energy or sports drinks or vitamin waters, the more prone they are to weight gain, diabetes and a whole host of ills. Even one can of soda a week increases the risk for gaining weight. In fact, weight increases for every 3 ounces of soda consumed, which is about three gulps of cola. Imagine what a can or bottle a day can do for your waistline and your mood!

Pop-a-holic

Could you drink 650 cans of soda? No? Well, most people can. Every man, woman and child in the United States averages 54 gallons of soda a year, or the equivalent of 650 cans. At 10 teaspoons of sugar per can, that's 106 teaspoons of sugar every week just from soda, and more than 49 pounds of sugar every year. Put another way, the average American is pouring ten 5-pound bags of sugar down his or her throat every year, just from soda. If you are like me, you don't waste your money on sugar water, which means someone is drinking your share. That's a whopping dose of nutritionally defunct sweetened junk and the number one source of sugar in our diets. Just cutting out bottled sugar-water drinks would make a huge dent in America's waistline.

From the first sip, soft drinks are ravaging the body—corroding tooth enamel, confusing appetite chemicals in the digestive tract, dissolving bone, filling fat cells and encouraging organ breakdown that leads to diabetes. Every time you have a soft drink, you are adding about 200 extra calories to your day's intake. Even if you had a measly can a week, that equates to a 3-pound weight gain over the course of one year. In fact, people who drink sugar-sweetened drinks—from soft drinks and bottled teas to sports waters and energy drinks—double their chances of being fat. From a global perspective, introduce soft drinks to a country and within no time obesity and diabetes rates skyrocket.

Even water can pack on the pounds. Fancy bottled water, that is. Waters with added vitamins, herbs and flavorings often replace good old tap water. Just because it's clear doesn't mean it's calorie free! Some vitamin waters supply the same calories as a cola. That's like having a scoop of vanilla ice cream on a waffle cone! The bottled teas, like the ones Sarah was drinking, unless they are artificially sweetened, add the same calories as you'd get in a side order of hash browns.

Think you're doing your heart good by drinking bottled tea? Think again. The antioxidant compounds in home-brewed tea that lower your risk for cancer and heart disease don't make it into the bottle. Tea is a great thirst quencher and perfect indulgence that boosts mood and helps you lose weight—just make it at home and skip the bottled stuff. (See Chapter 9 for more on how tea can help with weight loss and mood.)

What should you do?

- Skip soft drinks altogether, or drink diet versions of your favorite brands. Even then, limit intake to no more than one or two a week. Besides saving calories, your pocketbook will thank you for it. At about $1.50 a bottle, that daily sugar habit costs almost $550 a year!

- Never bring soft drinks into the home; save them for special occasions, such as a baseball game or a trip to the movies.

- Order water or nonfat milk with meals at restaurants.

- On rare occasions (i.e., once or twice a year) when you do order a soda, choose the smallest size and ask for extra ice.

- Save your money on the bottled energy drinks and vitamin waters. Instead, carry a water bottle from home.

- To make plain water more enticing, flavor it with fresh lemon slices or True Lemon powder.

Go for the Thick Liquids

Weight gain is only likely with calorific, clear liquids. Other drinks, especially thick liquids, like soups, smoothies or tomato juice, actually help with weight loss. That's because they fill us up so we eat less. Less food means less calories means more weight loss. Having a glass of tomato juice before a meal or a homemade smoothie in place of a meal is a trick many happy, fit people use to satisfy hunger and cut back on calories.

Beware of most store-bought smoothies. They typically are loaded with added sugar, up to 13 teaspoons
per bottle! They also might contain mood-lowering
saturated fats, like coconut milk, or questionable
ingredients like royal jelly or ginseng. Check the label
for serving size, too. That little bottle you think is
just one serving could be two, with twice the calories
and sugar. Even smoothies that look healthy can be
calorie-packed.

Instead, follow happy, fit people's advice and
quench your thirst with a smoothie made at home
from super mood foods like soy milk, berries and
oranges. Or drink 100% fruit juice, such as orange,
pineapple, grapefruit or tomato. Keep the serving size
to no more than 1 cup for juice and 2 cups (16 ounces)
for smoothies.

Here are some quick, easy recipes for super mood
smoothies:

- *Strawberry-Peach Smoothie:* Place strawberries
  and peeled peach slices in a blender, add
  nonfat plain yogurt, a tablespoon of orange
  juice concentrate and a handful of ice.
- *Chocolate-Berry Smoothie:* Place frozen
  raspberries, half a banana and chocolate soy
  milk in a blender.
- *Wake up and Smell the Coffee Smoothie:*
  Instead of coffee in the morning, place low-fat
  milk fortified with DHA, 2 teaspoons instant

coffee, one packet of vanilla flavored instant breakfast and three graham crackers in a blender.

- *PB&J Smoothie:* Place nonfat milk, low-fat cottage cheese, 2 tablespoons peanut butter, a small banana and 1 tablespoon honey in a blender.
- *Almondine Smoothie:* Place a nectarine (pit removed), 1 ounce of almonds, 1 tablespoon honey and ¼ teaspoon almond extract in a blender.

Is Fruit Juice Fattening?

Fruit juice is loaded with antioxidants, vitamins and minerals, as long as it is 100% juice and doesn't contain concentrated white grape, apple or pear juice. (These fruit concentrates are a way of adding processed sugar without having to put "sweetened with added sugar" on the label.) Juice doesn't have the fiber that whole fruit does, so it isn't as filling and the calories can add up if you overdo it. Also, some of the antioxidant-rich phytonutrients are lost when fruit skins and seeds are removed.

While whole fruit is best, juice is good for you, as long as it is 100% juice and the label doesn't contain the words *beverage, ade, cocktail, drink,* or *blend.* Cranberry juice helps reduce the risk for urinary tract infections. Orange juice lowers blood pressure. Pomegranate juice might lower total cholesterol levels. Your best bets include 100% orange juice, grapefruit juice, pineapple juice, prune juice and tomato juice. Limit daily intake to no more than 1 cup (8 ounces).

The Jitter Threshold

I worked with Sasha in Chicago for a *Good Morning America* segment on the mood-altering effects of coffee. Sasha lived on coffee, drinking up to five grandes a day. She swore she would crumble into a blithering, fatigued idiot without a constant caffeine dose. "I have a high-demand job and I barely have the energy I need to keep up the pace, even with coffee," she told me. She was convinced she couldn't survive without caffeine. Yet she agreed to wean herself off the brew, if only for the chance to be on national television. To avoid the deadly caffeine withdrawal headache, I asked her to first cut back by one grande a day. The next week, she cut back to three grandes and made one half decaffeinated. By the end of the third week, she was caffeine-free.

The results were amazing. Not only did Sasha not crumble into a heap from fatigue, she actually had more energy than when she had been living on coffee:

"My energy level has always fluctuated throughout the day. I'd feel energized, then exhausted. That's when I'd grab another coffee. But once I was weaned off caffeine, I found I had more energy and my energy level stayed consistently high all day long. I sleep better now and my mood has improved. I can't believe how much better I feel!"

Caffeine is a wolf in sheep's clothing. Yes, it is the jolt we need to start our engines in the morning, but it also fuels fatigue. By blocking a nerve chemical called adenosine, caffeine keeps our nervous system wide awake. It works its magic within minutes of making it into the bloodstream, leaving us less tired, more alert, better able to concentrate and faster to react. Just one small cup of coffee and people type faster and with more accuracy, drive better in rush-hour traffic, perform better on tests and show improved short-term memory.

The high is followed by a crash. The first sign of caffeine withdrawal is fatigue. Within an hour or two of the last cup (the time varies from one person to the next), a person feels tired, crabby, shaky, even depressed. Like Sasha, it is easy to return to the coffee for another pick-me-up, and the cycle continues.

"Caffeine lifts you out of a grumpy state, but drink too much and it actually contributes to depression," says Dr. Larry Christensen at the University of South Alabama, whose research found that some mood problems are fixed by eliminating caffeine. "We found in our studies on depression that even one week of going cold turkey on caffeine was enough to see a mood and energy improvement in about half of our subjects."

Try eliminating caffeine for two weeks and see if your mood or sleep patterns improve. After that, you can try adding back a cup or two a day, as long as it doesn't affect your mood. But refrain from a return to hourly trips to Starbucks!

Healthy Brew

Caffeine aside, coffee offers a few compelling health benefits for your body and mind that give java junkies reason to perk up. Coffee appears to lower the risk for heart disease and for dying from heart disease by up to 24%. The brew also helps lower the risk for certain cancers, such as colon, rectal and liver cancers. Something in coffee, other than caffeine, also lowers the risk for gout and diabetes and might protect against Parkinson's disease. Coffee also might keep you mentally sharp into your senior years and extend your life.

Coffee a health drink? Coffee is an extract, and like other extracts, including wine, cocoa and tea, it is packed with antioxidants that protect cells' genetic code or DNA from damage and promote cell survival. Coffee also might reduce inflammation associated with blood vessel damage. Of course, other studies have found that coffee might increase risks for pancreatic cancer and even might increase heart disease risk, so it is premature to recommend guzzling cup after cup every day. Also, how the coffee is made appears important to health, with filtered drip being healthier than pressed coffee.

Less Is More

Caffeine lingers in the body for hours. As a consequence, coffee drinkers take longer to fall asleep, sleep less soundly, wake up more often and wake up groggier than nonusers. A restless night, in turn, is likely to leave you dragging the next day, which is exactly what was happening to Sasha. Lack of sleep tips the scales in favor of weight gain, increasing the chances of packing on extra pounds by up to 70%!

Substituting a cup of tea or a diet Pepsi for an evening cup of coffee will not avoid insomnia, since both the tea and the Pepsi contain the same amount of caffeine as a cup of instant coffee. Finally, coffee acts as a diuretic, contributing to dehydration, which in turn causes fatigue. The irony is that, like Sasha, many people say they have more energy within weeks of giving up or at least cutting back on the very drink they thought was energizing them. (Check out Chapter 10 for more information on caffeine and sleep.)

You can have coffee without sacrificing your mood, sleep or waistline. Just limit intake to no more than three 8-ounce cups a day, and drink those in the early part of the day. Since caffeine can linger for up to 12 hours in the body, a latte at 4:00 p.m. could leave you tossing and turning at midnight. Also, make sure you aren't overdosing on calories with a beverage that should be calorie free.

Coffee Calories

Coffee is almost calorie free, so it is a great substitute for dessert at the end of a meal, as long as it is decaffeinated! But start adding whipped cream, whole milk, chocolate syrups and other goodies and you chalk up more fat and calories than a big slice of cheesecake. For example, top any gourmet coffee drink with whipped cream and you've added 110 calories of fat. If consumed daily, that's enough to produce a 1-pound weight gain each month. Even if you only have a whipped-topped coffee once a week, you still could gain almost 2 pounds over the course of a year.

From mochas to frappuccinos, gourmet coffee drinks are usually a combination of coffee, sweetened milk, ice and syrups. They range in calories from 120 calories to 500, depending on how much chocolate and flavored syrups, the type of milk and how big they are. For example,

- A café mocha made with whole milk contains up to 400 calories and almost 7 teaspoons of fat, beating out chocolate fudge cake by 150 calories! Add a dollop of whipped cream and the calories jump to more than 500 and you've used up 60% of your daily allotment for fat, or more than 40 grams.
- Order a Dunkin' Donuts Hazelnut Coolata and you'll be downing a 370-calorie drink with 5 teaspoons of fat, which is like having a hot fudge sundae with nuts.
- Top your latte with whipped cream and grated milk chocolate and you're sipping more calories and fat than a ½ cup of Häagen-Dazs butter pecan ice cream (or about 350 calories and 20 grams of fat).

You can have your latte and drink it, too, just tweak the ingredients.

- Sprinkle your mochas lightly with cinnamon and cocoa powder for low-fat flavor, and just say "no" to the whipped cream and chocolate shavings.
- Order an espresso with a twist of lemon for a no-calorie jolt of coffee reality.
- Think of your coffee drink as your dessert for the day and have the whipped cream and chocolate shavings, then "just say no" to the ice cream that night.

Liquor Is Quicker

While a glass of wine is one of life's little pleasures, too much alcohol can be a dieter's nemesis. It is calorie dense, more fattening than food and dissolves our resolve to eat right.

I'll Have a Quarter Pounder in a Glass, Please

Alcohol is the least filling of the four calorie-containing substances. (Protein is the most filling, followed by carbs, then fat, and finally alcohol.) At 7 calories a gram, alcohol has a calorie content closest to fat. It doesn't take a math wizard to see that the calories add up fast. The average drink, such as a beer, glass of wine or shot of liquor, supplies about 150 calories, but that's just a start. Add sugary mixes or cream to any drink and the calories double or even triple.

You also are probably getting more than you realize. In one study, researchers visited 80 bars and restaurants and found that bartenders were pouring up to 50% larger drinks than the recommended serving size. That means people who follow the guidelines to limit intake to one drink a day may be getting more than they bargained for—more alcohol *and* more calories.

We often think of beer as fattening, but you'll gain weight twice as fast on a Lemon Drop or tall rum & Coke as on a can of beer. A large margarita supplies about 450 calories (the calorie equivalent of 18 chocolate Kisses), and a tall Long Island Iced Tea has up to 1,000 calories (the calorie equivalent of a platter of fried onion rings). An apple martini can pack up to 350 calories, depending on the recipe. You probably wouldn't dream of eating a big slice of chocolate cake with butter-fudge frosting before dinner, but you've just gulped the equivalent in calories in that one drink alone. If you were to have two apple martinis and a beer at happy hour, you would be gulping more calories than is in two Quarter Pounders! You also are more likely to overindulge when at a bar, since the loud noise encourages you to drink more and faster.

Alcohol Is Really Fattening

Not all calories are created equal. Unlike protein, carbs and healthy fats, which are essential nutrients, alcohol is toxic. It damages tissues, destroys cells and interferes with organ function. For this reason, the body has evolved a complex system to rid itself of alcohol as fast as possible. It "burns" alcohol calories first and stores other calories coming in from food as body fat. So the fat in a Kahlua and cream, in the butter on bread, or in the fettuccini alfredo accompanying a glass of wine, which in the absence of alcohol might be burned for energy, heads straight for storage on the thighs, hips and waist. As a result, a meal that includes alcohol is much more fattening than any other meal, because the alcohol has added extra calories to the meal *and* every calorie from the food in excess of the body's immediate needs is stored as fat.

It Dissolves Our Resolve

Not only does alcohol add calories, it also entices us to eat more. It stimulates our appetite and crumbles our diet guard. In fact, we gobble up to 200 more calories when a meal is accompanied by one alcoholic drink than when we don't imbibe. Nighttime drinking is the worst, since it is highly unlikely you'll head from the bar to the gym to work off the calories, so the calories are stacked on top of your total day's intake.

That's what happened to James, an attorney in Encinitas, California:

"I attend a lot of business-related events in the evening. I vow before each engagement to steer clear of the buffet table or just snack on broccoli.

But once I have a drink in my hand, it's like I'm possessed by the grease demon. I'll power down fistfuls of chips and dip or a plateload of potato skips heaped with cheese and bacon."

The thousands of calories noshed standing up were enough to cause James's cholesterol to soar and his waistline to bulge. When he started ordering diet cola with a twist at these events, he also regained control of his appetite. "No one even knew I wasn't drinking, they thought I'd switched to bourbon and soda. I lost 25 pounds. Better yet, by staying sober, I've learned so much more about my colleagues and clients!"

Eating a little extra is not a problem if a person only has a glass or two of wine a week, but Americans average 2.5 gallons of alcohol a year—or two to five drinks a day. We drink to have fun. We drink to relax. We drink to indulge ourselves, to celebrate and to bond with friends. Don't get me wrong. It's fine to include a little alcohol in our lives. It might even boost health, reduce our risk for disease and extend our lives (see Chapter 9). But this habit also could undermine your mood and widen your waistline if you are not careful.

Cheers to Your Health

A little alcohol is good for you, or at least it's good for your heart. It keeps the arteries clear, dissolves blood clots that can otherwise lodge in arteries leading to heart attack and stroke, and gives the good type of cholesterol, called HDL, a little boost. Moderate drinking also might reduce the risk for dementia and vision loss in later years.

Drink too much, though, and the damage far outweighs the bonuses in terms of your health, mood and quality of life. Excessive drinking destroys your body and leaves you crabby, depressed, forgetful, sleep deprived and fatigued. One study found that while a drink a day reduced the risk for dementia later in life, more than two drinks a day doubled the risk. It also can leave you dead if you do something stupid like drink and drive.

Drink too much and you also mess up your nutrition by flushing mood-boosting nutrients out of the body, like vitamin C, potassium and calcium, as well as magnesium, zinc, vitamin A and the B vitamins. Any or all of those deficiencies will leave you mentally muddled, down in the dumps and too pooped to enjoy life.

Anyone with at least two functioning brain cells knows you shouldn't mix alcohol and medications, both prescription and over-the-counter. Alcohol can enhance a drug's action, leading to greater side effects. It can cancel out or lessen a medication's effectiveness, such as in the case of antibiotics. Alcohol can convert medications to toxic chemicals that damage tissues (e.g., mixing alcohol with Tylenol can cause liver damage). Finally, alcohol can magnify the sedative effects of certain medications, including antidepressants.

What's Too Much?

It's easy to spot a drunk, right? They drink until they are sloppy drunk. They may have a history of drunk driving or have had blackouts where they can't remember what they did the night before. They might have a drink in the morning to relieve a hangover. Those are the blaring signs. More often than not, however, the signs are more subtle.

How can you tell if you drink too much? By answering this question: is it interfering with my life, job, social and family relationships or health? If anyone is having a problem with your drinking, then it's a problem. General guidelines for defining the terms are

A light drinker: No more than three drinks a week (one drink = one 12-ounce beer, a 5-ounce glass of wine or 1 ounce hard liquor)

A moderate drinker: No more than 13 drinks a week, and no more than two drinks on most days of the week

A heavy drinker: Has 14 or more drinks a week, or more than two drinks almost every day

---

The Best Thirst Quenchers

A can of diet pop, a glass of wine or an energy drink a few times a week is fine. But if you find you are drinking closer to the average in this country—a gallon of sugar-filled canned or bottled drinks a week and/or more than one alcoholic beverage every day—then you have ventured outside the thirst-quenching boundary of what happy, fit people have found works for their moods and waistlines.

Moderation is the key. Soft drinks should be an occasional treat, not a daily habit. Have one or two a month, not a day. To maximize the health benefits of alcohol, such as lowering heart disease risk, and to avoid the dangers of weight gain and depression, most happy, fit people limit alcohol to one drink a day or less.

Have your glass of wine with rather than before, between or after meals. A glass of wine with a healthy meal that includes soup, salad, vegetables, lean meat and fruit for dessert combines the ingredients needed to enhance feeling full on fewer calories. On the other hand, drink during happy hour and you're more likely to munch on a ton of greasy appetizers.

Who Sails Your Vessel?

You have vowed either to not drink alcohol or sugary drinks or to drink in moderation. Sometimes that is easier said than done. Most people don't like to drink alone, so the social pressure to join the crowd can be stiff. Toasting the birthday boy or ringing in the New Year doesn't have to mean drinking alcohol at all and certainly doesn't require getting drunk. Just because everyone else orders a soft drink or a martini at the restaurant, doesn't mean you should do the same. But what do you do if the only beverage offered is soda or beer?

One habit worth practicing is planning ahead of time how you will handle these key situations when the pressure or temptation to drink the wrong stuff can overwhelm your best intentions to break this habit. That plan might include

- **Serve nonalcoholic and sugar-free alternatives at parties and social events.** Bring your own to someone else's party.
- **Pace your drinking.** Plan to alternate one glass of wine or soda with a glass of water, or dilute a drink with lots of water, fruit juice or ice.
- **Think light.** Do your waistline a big favor and switch from regular beer to non-alcoholic beer. You will cut calories in half. Check labels on light beers, since they vary in calorie content, so you will save lots—or next to no—calories, depending on the brand.
- **Nix the drinks made with high-calorie mixes.** Make your one alcoholic drink a day a glass of wine and you'll save a hundred or more calories.
- **Dress up nonalcoholic drinks.** Add zest to club soda, diet ginger ale or other drinks by serving them in fancy glasses garnished with straws and fruit wedges.
- **Think grapes, not wine.** Make nonalcoholic drinks with purple or red grape juice to get some of the health-boosting compounds found in red wine. Look for concord grape juice that has not

been diluted with white grape juice. Other foods that contain heart-healthy compounds found in red wine include berries, plums, currants, all deep red-blue fruits, apples, onions, oranges and grapefruit.

- **Eat well.** Keep healthful snacks handy so you have something else to do with your hands and mouth besides gulp down another drink.
- **Drink water, not soda pop, to quench your thirst.** The best rule of all.

Water: The Perfect Beverage

Water is the perfect beverage. It is fat free, sugar free and calorie free, and it works with, rather than against, our bodies' natural thirst and hunger systems. Replace the typical 19 ounces of soft drinks, energy drinks, vitamin waters or bottled teas guzzled daily by each American with plain water and you will quench your thirst and cut almost 250 calories from your daily diet, the equivalent of a 1-pound weight loss every two weeks, or 26 pounds in a year.

Water always has been and always will be the most important nutrient in our diets. Second only to oxygen, it is absolutely critical for life. We need water for almost all body functions, including digestion, absorption, circulation, excretion, transporting nutrients, building tissue and maintaining body temperature. Everything in the body—from reproduction to mood and memory—depends on water. Water helps ward off fatigue (the number one health complaint in the United States), keeps tissues hydrated and helps prevent headaches, kidney stones and urinary tract infections. It even helps make us smarter, wards off memory loss and improves attention.

In short, your body just won't work right without enough water. It can't rid itself of waste products, so toxins accumulate. The cells can't function properly when water balance is disrupted. Even mild dehydration, such as losing 1% to 2% of body weight or 1½ pounds for a 150-pound person, results in a variety of problems, from headaches, fatigue and weakness to lightheadedness, poor stamina, reduced short-term memory and poor concentration and reasoning ability.

Hungry or Thirsty?

The next time you find yourself tempted to nibble on something sinful, like chips, try drinking a glass of water and waiting 15 minutes to see if the urge to snack subsides.

Why? Some people aren't in tune with their hunger signals and mistake hunger for thirst, turning to ice cream when what their bodies really want is a glass of ice water. In one study, two out of every three people who had lost weight and maintained the weight loss said they "make a concerted effort to drink water to control their weight." It tastes good, is refreshing and helps them limit the amount they eat. Happy, fit people also say that drinking a glass of water helps them satisfy the desire to eat between meals when they aren't really hungry; they just need something to sip on, rather than something to nosh.

The 8x8 Rule

You can't go a day without replenishing your body's water supply. Hey, we aren't camels! Our bodies can't store excess water for future times of need. What goes out must be replaced ASAP. That means daily intakes are essential, preferably spread evenly throughout the day, not gulped all at one time. Your body processes water slowly. Drink a quarter cup of water every 15 minutes and it has time to make it into tissues. Drink a quart in five minutes and most of the water will be flushed out in the urine.

Follow the 8x8 rule: drink at least eight 8-ounce glasses of water a day. That's about how much fluid your body loses just staying alive. Of course, that's just a guideline and some people will need more than the basic 8x8, including people who exercise, live or work in hot climates or perspire heavily and women who are pregnant or breast-feeding.

The bottom line: you need at least eight glasses, every day, seven days a week, preferably sipped rather than gulped.

You'll know if you are getting enough fluid when

your urine is pale yellow to clear and you urinate every two to four hours. Dark yellow urine is a sign your body is lacking in water and is trying to conserve. (One exception to this rule is if you take large doses of B vitamins, which can color the urine a bright yellow.)

Water Bottle Blues

Reusable bottles, some baby bottles, plastic utensils and many clear plastic food-storage containers contain an estrogen-like chemical called bisphenol-A (BPA) that has been linked to cancer, heart disease, diabetes, altered thyroid function, enlarged prostates and abnormal development of reproductive organs, at least in animals. BPA also could have damaging effects on infant brain and nerve development. Even in amounts considered "safe" by the Environmental Protection Agency, BPA might impair brain function—again at least in animals. Hot liquids and food enhance leaching in BPA-containing plastics. For example, boiling water increases leaching up to fifty-five-fold. It is assumed that microwaving in these containers also is dangerous.

The worrisome issue is that a study from the Centers for Disease Control and Prevention found that 95% of people screened tested positive for BPA. The research is so convincing that some countries, like Canada, are taking steps to ban BPA from all products. Currently, manufacturers are not required to label BPA on containers, so there is no way to identify which plastics contain the potentially dangerous chemical. The best alternative is to use stainless steel, glass or plastics labeled "BPA-free."

SECRET 9:
INDULGE IN THE RIGHT VICES

The Promise

In three weeks of making this change, you will:

- notice a reduction in cravings

In six months, you will:

- drop a few pounds
- have an easier time sticking with your weight-loss plans
- feel more relaxed and your cravings will be mild, if at all

In one year, you will:

- be in control of your vices and cravings
- lower your risk for diseases, such as heart disease, cancer and dementia

Vices. We all have them. We wouldn't be human if we didn't! Some vices are just plain naughty, like smoking, which is a death sentence at almost any dose. Other vices, such as drinking alcohol, gambling or eating sweets, straddle the fence between naughty and nice, depending on how often and how much we indulge. A few vices, like red wine, tea and chocolate, are actually mood-boosting, waist-thinning, disease-preventing, life-extending wonders—as long as we stay within limits.

The "vice" of food cravings is not a sign of a split personality or even a lack of willpower. You aren't a bad person because you can't keep your hands out of the cookie jar or spoon out of the ice cream. More often than not, those cravings are fueled by a whole symphony of brain chemicals; other times it's just a habit—one that is easily tamed.

Fantastic Voyage

Vices aren't just learned, they are hardwired into your head. Serotonin, endorphins, neuropeptide Y (NPY), galanin and corticosterone might sound like characters from *Star Wars*, but they are some of the many microscopic chemicals at the helm of your craving control.

Some of these nerve chemicals originate from the brain's appetite control tower, the hypothalamus. Others are produced in satellite relay stations, such as the digestive tract, pancreas or the adrenal glands, that send detailed messages to the brain. Some switch on the desire to eat sweet or fatty foods; others tell us when to stop. Each of us rides the ebb and flow of these chemicals.

The most famous of all brain chemicals is serotonin, which, when levels get low in the brain, turns on a craving for carbs and drops mood into the blue-and-gloomy range. Give in to the craving by eating a piece of pie or an oatmeal cookie and the brain rapidly makes more serotonin, which then triggers a better mood and a drop in cravings. That's why so many people return over and over again to sweets to feel good. Winnie, a government worker in Milwaukee, says, "My best friend is a Cinnabon roll. I can always count on it to brighten my day when I'm feeling sorry for myself." Too bad that roll also has 730 calories, enough to explain why Winnie gained 15 pounds in one year.

But that's just one of many chemicals coursing through your brain and body sending subtle, unconscious reminders that you deserve another chip or would feel so much better if you just had a chocolate Kiss. NPY tells you to include carbs at breakfast. By lunch, a brain chemical called galanin is telling you to eat fattier fare. During times of stress, it might be the endorphins released into your brain telling you that something sweet and creamy right now sure would taste good. These nerve chemicals are ebbing and flowing throughout the day, throughout the month and even throughout the year, leading to cravings for salty popcorn during the winter months, ice cream just before a woman's period and pancakes for breakfast year-round.

The Natural High

Indulging in small amounts of good vices can keep you on the diet track and even boost your mood while losing weight.

A Closer Look at the Sweet and Creamies

Sweets mean sugar, right? Not always. In fact, most sweets are more fat than carbs. Our favorite vices typically are a combination of sugar and fat. We are after the sweet, but it is the fat that draws us in and can add inches to our waistlines. For example, well over 50% of the calories in most ice creams and 40% or more of the calories in a chocolate chip cookie come from fat, not sugar.

Fat alone is unpalatable—who craves a big glob of lard? But add even a little sugar and it becomes a sweet-and-creamy combination that brings out the craving in even the most ardent dieter. Sugar makes fat taste good and even masks its presence in foods.

When people taste foods containing various amounts of sugar and fat, their perception of the fat content decreases as the sugar content increases; the sweeter the treat, the more we don't taste the fat. Sugar makes the fat invisible. Consequently, people often have no idea how much fat they are eating and unjustly accuse only sugar of prompting the uncontrollable urge to eat—and the spare tire around the middle.

Serotonin definitely leads us to crave sweets, but don't put all the blame on serotonin for your sweet-and-creamy cravings. More likely, it is serotonin working in concert with endorphins—natural morphine-like substances in the brain—that produce euphoric or pleasurable feelings whenever you take a bite of whipped cream–topped pie or a hot fudge sundae. Both sugar and fat release endorphins in the brain and produce a natural painkilling effect. In fact, the very taste of sugar on the tongue releases endorphins in the brain. That means that you start feeling happy as soon as something sweet hits your tongue. No wonder chocolate, the ultimate melt-in-your-mouth combination of fat and sugar, is the number one most craved food.

Basic Instincts

The desire to eat forbidden fruits, from Indian fry bread to Ben & Jerry's, might spring from an even deeper internal well than a craving for pleasure or even a relief from depression or boredom.

It is no coincidence that the appetite control center in the brain is next door to the reproductive center, which leads many researchers to suspect that the cycle of fat and sugar cravings coincides with reproductive needs, otherwise known as the survival of the species instinct.

Your most basic driving force is to survive, and nothing is more important to that drive than making sure the body has enough to eat. It's no surprise that all the appetite control chemicals in the brain turn on cravings for high-calorie sweets and grease; there are no brain chemicals—not one—that whisper in your inner ear to eat broccoli or wheat germ (unless the broccoli is battered and fried or the wheat germ is disguised in cookie batter!). Sweet and greasy foods were rare on the savannah during most of our ancient ancestor's Stone Age lives. Over millions of years, these ancestors evolved complicated brain chemistry to ensure they ate anything with lots of calories whenever it happened to show up, just to make sure they survived the next famine.

Perhaps that very basic survival drive explains why women battle more cravings than do men and are more likely to crave sweetened fats, especially during puberty and following ovulation. Cravings are the body's way of making sure that women's hips have packed on ample calories to get them through pregnancy, birthing and nursing the next generation.

Men, on the other hand, typically prefer protein fats, such as meat dishes, perhaps as a survival instinct that ensures they have the muscle and fortitude to bring home the bacon (or bison, as the case may be) for their families.

Stress adds to the craving equation. Everything from boredom to anxiety can set off a craving attack. Interestingly, the stress hormones, such as norepinephrine (a cousin to adrenaline) and corticosterone, both made and released from the adrenal glands during stress, raise brain levels of appetite control chemicals, which in turn increase food cravings, overeating and weight gain. Which makes sense from a survival-of-the-fittest perspective.

Of course, these survival skills and the cravings they trigger don't suit our modern-day madness, where sweet and greasy treats have gone from few to frequent and tigers have been replaced with deadlines. But our bodies are identical to our ancestors' cave-dweller bodies, and those bodies evolved to literally kill for a cookie (or anything high in fat, sugar and calories).

Work with Them, Not Against Them

You can't will away food cravings; they are part of the human package. Restrictive diets or even very low-fat or carb-free diets disrupt this natural cycle of nerve chemicals. These nerve chemicals go totally berserk when people go on quick-weight loss diets, since those diets try to force our appetites to go against everything they evolved to do. The more a person diets, the more out of control the cravings.

People who repeatedly gain and lose weight on fad diets also crave sweet-fat foods more than do people who lose weight sensibly and for good. It is likely that restricting these foods raises some appetite chemicals and lowers others, which sets up a rebound effect and swings the eating pendulum from abstinence to binge. You can't get mad at those chemicals, they are only doing their job—ensuring you stay alive.

Don't get me wrong. I'm not giving you license to binge on junk. You must find a happy medium between including a few vices in your day without those cravings running your life and jeopardizing your waistline or your health. The secret to being happier and skinnier is to work with your appetite control chemicals, not against them. Ask any happy person who has maintained a desirable weight for any length of time and you'll find that most, if not all of them, indulge their vices now and then.

10 Steps to Crave Control

Whatever the cause, the only solution is to work with the cravings, not try to will them away. Happy, fit people have different ways of doing this:

- Darlene, the teacher in Albuquerque, found she could keep her sugar cravings at bay by eating protein: "I pack string cheese sticks in my purse or briefcase or toss a handful of peanuts into my mouth whenever I'm hit with the urge to snack. That usually is all it takes to calm the craving storm."

- Rainey, a speaker's bureau consultant in Washington, D.C., follows the "if...then" rule. "My philosophy is that if I want a glass of red wine (which I usually do these days), then I will not have anything white that day, like white bread or rice." She's also found that having a big bowl of fruit after dinner helps curb her sweet tooth and keeps her out of the ice cream.

- Reka, who works at a publishing house in New York, says, "When it comes to vices, I like them all—sweet, salty, greasy, you name it. What I've found that works for me when a craving hits is to put a big bowl of baby carrots on my desk at work. It gives me something to crunch on and I can eat as many as I want without feeling guilty."

Diet is not shaped by food cravings alone. Along with that ancient brain telling you to eat sweets and fat, you have a higher brain, called the cortex, that can keep you on track dietwise. Eating right means engaging that cortex to adopt a willing attitude and a bit of up-front planning.

Controlling your vices begins with 10 simple steps:

1. *Eat regularly.* You stay in control of your appetite and cravings if you eat frequently, starting with breakfast. You stay in control of your cravings when you are comfortably hungry. Let more than four hours go by between meals or snacks and you could be too hungry to make smart decisions. Now your cravings control you, setting the stage for an out-of-control binge.

2. *Ride the wave.* Just because you have a hankering for a bag of corn chips doesn't mean you give in to the craving immediately. Make a rule that you will ride the crave wave for at least 20 minutes, then if you still want the chip, have it. Or tell yourself you'll have that snack tomorrow. Often telling yourself you can have something "later," rather than "never," is enough to soothe the urge.

While you are riding the crave wave, try chewing gum. Studies show that popping a stick of gum in your mouth can reduce cravings, suppress appetite, reduce your desire for sweets and help you cut back on snacking.

3. *Plan your cravings.* Set aside a calorie allotment to accommodate a small indulgence a few times a week. Then have whatever you want, just limit it to three bites. That's all it takes to satisfy your brain chemistry. Besides, research shows that the most enjoyment comes in the first bite. Each subsequent bite becomes less and less enjoyable and more and more like a binge.

4. *Out of sight.* Hide your temptations, if you bring them into the house at all. Out of sight often really does mean out of mind.

5. *Repackage it.* Overdoing it is easy when you eat straight from the bag of chips or carton of ice cream. Portion dry snacks into 1-ounce servings and place in baggies. Scoop the recommended half-cup serving of ice cream into a bowl and put the carton back in the freezer before eating it. Susan, a mother and executive in Southern California, learned to satisfy her cravings with a small bite of something sweet after every meal. "I've always craved something sweet after lunch and dinner. So I made myself a bargain. I could have two Milk Duds or one piece of licorice after every lunch and dinner. That satisfies the craving. Any more than that, and I feel terrible, probably from guilt." Hey, if you're going to feel guilty, why not use it in your favor?

6. *Find a better way.* Find a healthier option for each craving. Need something crunchy and creamy? Try dunking baby carrots in peanut butter. Need a sweet, crunchy alternative to a Snickers bar? Try dates stuffed with almonds. Is sweet and creamy your weakness? Try custard-style yogurt topped with a dollop of light whipped cream.

*7. **You deserve the best.*** Don't "waist" your calories on low-quality sweets. Skip the boxed cookies, the commercial doughnuts and the cheap candy bars. Instead, when you decide to indulge, pick the best of the best. A small piece of high-quality chocolate will satisfy you far more than a pound of junk.

*8. **Keep a journal.*** For one week, write down everything you eat and how you feel before and after. You might find that certain emotions, people, places or events trigger cravings. Once you figure out the link, it's easy to find a solution.

*9. **Is it only a habit?*** Often we program ourselves to crave a food. Have a bite of chocolate after lunch, and before you know it, you must have chocolate after every meal. Habits are learned, so they can be unlearned. In this case, develop a new habit that provides the same pleasurable or rewarding effect. For example, take a brisk walk, shoot baskets, call a friend, paint your nails or take a hot bath during that craving-prone time of the day.

*10. **Get moving.*** People who are physically active are less prone to bingeing and cravings and maintain a more constant weight as compared to couch potatoes. Exercise also is a healthy way to get a pleasurable endorphin rush and reduce stress. The best part is that when you exercise daily and vigorously, you can indulge a little more in your vices! Understanding that food cravings are fueled not just by personality, but by a stew of nerve chemicals and hormones takes the guilt out of cravings and helps you work with and listen to your body. Besides, some vices are good for us. We need a little decadence in our lives to boost our spirits and tantalize our tastebuds. More important, some vices actually lower disease risk, extend the healthy years and even improve mood, memory and weight. If you are going to indulge, do it with a delicious treat that makes you happy and smart, like tea, wine or chocolate. All three of these foods have one thing in common—they are extracts, which are condensed versions of antioxidant-rich plants. It makes sense that they are absolutely good-for-you vices.

30 Indulgences That Will Soothe Any Craving

1. **Mango Parfait:** Layer cubes of mango, grated lemon zest and Rachel's Orange Strawberry Mango yogurt in a parfait glass. Top with a dollop of light whipped cream.

2. **Angel Food Cake à la Blueberries:** In a saucepan, heat 1 cup blueberries (fresh or frozen) with 1 tablespoon sugar or Splenda and 1 tablespoon cornstarch until sauce thickens. Let cool. Top a slice of angel food cake with the sauce.

3. **Grilled Pineapple:** Spray grill with cooking spray. Brush strips of fresh pineapple with rum and place on grill. Grill on each side until heated through, about three minutes per side. Top with toasted sweetened coconut.

4. **Poached Pear in Chocolate Lavender Sauce:** See recipe in Recipes section.

5. **Mini Chocolate Cream Pies:** Fill mini phyllo shells with cooled chocolate pudding (made with low-fat milk). Top with a dollop of fat-free whipped cream.

6. **Ice Cream Sandwiches:** Soften Breyer's Nonfat Double Churn-free Cappuccino Chocolate Chunk ice cream. Place a tablespoon between two chocolate wafers.

7. **Chocolate Fondue:** Melt semisweet chocolate pieces. Lightly dunk 1 cup fresh whole strawberries in the sauce.

8. **Fruit Kabobs:** Marinate nectarine or peach halves in lime juice, honey and concentrated orange juice. Thread skewers through fruit and grill.

9. **Trail Mix:** Mix equal parts tart dried cherries, almonds and semisweet chocolate chips. Limit serving to 2 ounces.

10. **Chewy, Crunchy, Super Chocolatey Clusters:** See recipe in Recipes section. Eat just one a day.

11. **Berry Cream:** Toss fresh berries with vanilla sugar. Place in wineglasses and top with a dollop of nonfat sour cream.

12. **Baked Apple:** Cut off the top of an apple and core. Sprinkle walnuts and brown sugar on top and bake at 375 degrees until tender, approximately 45 minutes.

13. **Sweet 'n' Creamy:** Top Rachel's Pink Grapefruit Lychee yogurt with blueberries.

14. **Bobbing for Apples:** Dunk apple slices in caramel sauce.

15. **Pineapple Coconut Smoothie:** See recipe in Recipes section.

16. **A Glass of Chocolate Satin:** Chocolate soy milk goes a long way to satisfying a chocolate craving!

17. **Cherry Jubilee:** Warm pitted cherries in the microwave and top with fat-free ricotta cheese and slivered almonds. Sprinkle with nutmeg.

18. **My Oh My Clementine:** Peel and section two clementine oranges. Top with warmed honey, crystalline ginger and ground cardamom.

19. **Chocolate Mousse:** Yoplait Whips Chocolate Mousse Style Yogurt topped with a sprinkling of semisweet chocolate chips and a dollop of fat-free whipped topping.

20. **Mango-Pineapple Crush:** See recipe in Recipes section.

21. **Sweet Cheeses:** Top graham crackers with fat-free ricotta cheese and strawberry jam or orange marmalade.

22. **Instant Pudding:** Top one prepared low-fat vanilla pudding snack cup with chopped pecans and diced dried apricots.

23. **Minty Fruit Sundae:** Blend nonfat plain yogurt with chopped fresh mint, vanilla extract and a touch of sugar. Pour over fresh fruit.

24. **Fooled Ya Ambrosia:** Mix pineapple chunks, banana slices, drained canned mandarin orange slices, nonfat vanilla yogurt, minimarshmallows and chopped walnuts in a bowl.

25. **Creamy, Spicy Crackers:** Top 100% whole-grain crackers with fat-free cream cheese and a dollop of jelly, such as red pepper jelly.

26. **Dessert on Toast:** Top a piece of whole-wheat toast with a thin smear of peanut butter, fat-free cottage cheese and drained crushed pineapple.

27. **Cookie Crumble:** Crush chocolate wafers and sprinkle over fat-free ricotta cheese.

28. **Spicy Chocolate Bruschetta:** Toast thin slices of a French baguette loaf. Melt semisweet chocolate with a touch of cayenne pepper in a pan. Top each slice with a little melted chocolate and orange shavings.

29. **Berry Frozen Yogurt Pie:** Soften a half gallon of fat-free vanilla frozen yogurt. Spoon into a graham cracker pie crust. Place in freezer until firm. Top each slice with ½ cup berries.

30. **Sweet Fruit McMuffins:** Cut a leftover dinner biscuit in half. Fill with fat-free sour cream and a teaspoon of jam. Top with fresh fruit.

The Tea Diet

There are only two ways to lose weight. You either 1. burn more calories or 2. eat fewer of them. Tea might help you do both.

First, compounds in tea called catechins rev metabolism and spark fat burning, so you burn more calories. Those calories are most likely to be fat calories from around your belly, hips and thighs. A few cups of tea each day raise your metabolism enough to burn about 80 extra calories. While it doesn't sound like much, over the course of a year that could mean up to an 8-pound loss, and all you did was sip on cups of tea! (Of course, that calorie advantage is shot if you more than make up the difference by eating more cookies.)

Second, a few studies show that drinking tea helps curb appetite, so you eat less. Maybe tea curbs your desire to gorge because drinking it gives you something to do, so you are less likely to circle the kitchen like a vulture, nibbling on everything from leftover Chinese take-out to crackers, cream cheese and pickles. Or it could be that tea's magic combination of caffeine and catechins, especially one called EGCG (which stands for epigallocatechin) is a one-two punch to your appetite-suppressing center.

Tea Time for Your Mood

As if being a natural diet aid wasn't enough, tea also has all the same benefits as coffee on your mood, without the downside of caffeine jitters. Since it has half the caffeine of coffee, or about 40 milligrams per cup (depending on how dark you like your brew), tea helps lift your spirits, speed thought processes and keep you energized but is less likely to interfere with a good night's sleep. Tea also helps soothe jangled nerves and lower stress. One study of healthy men found that those who drank tea had lower stress hormone levels and were more relaxed even when under pressure.

The Chinese believe that tea promotes health and longevity. They might be right. Tea is a gold mine of antioxidants that repair damaged cells in the brain and body. Other compounds in tea help relax arteries to encourage blood flow, reduce blood clots and prevent inflammation. The antioxidant load is so high in tea that when researchers at Tufts University compared it to antioxidants in 22 vegetables, tea came out on top as the best source of these cell-protecting compounds, with antioxidants that are more powerful than vitamin C, vitamin E or beta-carotene.

Improved blood flow and high antioxidants are the perfect combination for supplying oxygen and nutrients to your brain while protecting that delicate tissue from aging. No wonder people who drink tea are least likely to develop memory loss. The more tea they drink, the lower their risk for dementia. They also lower their risks for heart disease, cancer, osteoporosis and kidney stones.

Tea Rules

Green tea has received the most attention in the news when it comes to health and dieting. In reality, green, red (oolong), white and black teas all come from the same plant, whether it's grown in South America, Africa or Turkey. Granted, the leaves of green, red and black teas are processed differently and, yes, green tea has a ton of antioxidants, but so do red and black teas. White tea contains more of the buds and fewer of the leaves, but is still rich in antioxidants. Herb tea, on the other hand, has no relation to regular tea—the two come from totally different plants with totally different tastes, aromas and health benefits.

How much do you need? Ask an Irishman, and he might say to steep your tea until it is "strong enough for a mouse to trot on." That's probably overkill, especially for the mouse. A more reasonable goal is two to five cups a day, steeped for three to five minutes each. That gives you the antioxidant equivalent of one to two servings of vegetables (without all the healthy fiber, vitamins and minerals, of course). You get the biggest health benefits when you drink tea throughout life, not just for a few days.

Thinking about buying your tea premade? Big mistake. Bottled teas are basically just sugar water. All or almost all the antioxidants in the original tea are lost during processing and storage, since glass bottles expose the sensitive chemicals in tea, called flavonoids, to light. Instant powdered teas aren't much better and the process of decaffeinating teas destroys at least some of the antioxidants. Don't waste your money on tea extracts, pills or tablets, either.

Your best bet is also the cheapest—brew tea at home. Or get creative and try including tea in cooking, such as adding tea leaves or brew to rice puddings, homemade ice cream, scones or the Nutty Green Tea Rice in the Recipes section.

Grape Expectations

"I can't imagine life without wine," says Jeanette, a nurse in Salem, Oregon. "It is the one vice I'm totally not willing to give up. I don't care whether it's good, bad or indifferent to my health and waistline." Good thing Jeanette's chosen the right vice. This one is a great big plus for health—that is, when enjoyed in moderation.

Wine, red wine in particular, is like the proverbial apple a day in keeping the doctor away. It contains a slew of health-boosting, antioxidant-rich compounds, such as phenols, flavonoids, ergothionine and resveratrol, that protects arteries from inflammation and damage, lower heart disease risk and even prevent strokes and heart attacks. Wine and its stew of antioxidants also might lower the risk for dementia and even extend life. One study found that people who drank a moderate amount of wine were 40% less likely to become forgetful as they aged compared to teetotalers, while those drinking hard liquor increased their dementia risk.

What about white wine, is it good for you, too? Red wine contains at least 20 times the antioxidants of white wine (that's because the antioxidants are in the grape skin and red wine is processed with the skins, while white wine isn't). But white wine does have its virtues. White wine might improve your health, according to a study from the State University of New York, where researchers found that white wine, not red, improved breathing and lung function in a group of 1,555 adults. Lung function is a strong predictor of heart health, so toast to your lung and heart with a glass of Chablis!

As discussed in Chapter 8, you need to use some common sense when it comes to drinking any alcohol. All those antioxidants will do little for your mental health if you're rotting your liver with the toxic effects of too much alcohol. Women should limit their intake to one glass of wine, and men should cut themselves off at two glasses a day.

Wine Rules

For some of us, like Jeanette, life just isn't worth living without a vice or two, like a glass of wine or a nibble of chocolate. You also can make the vice work for you, your waistline and your mood, like Nancy, a freelance writer in Los Angeles, did:

"I joined Weight Watchers to relearn how to eat well. I'm on the Flex Plan, the one where you count your daily food points. The idea is to eat as much food as possible for the lowest possible points, which means lots of veggies. One thing that I must have, even though it amounts to 20% of my daily 20 points, is my nightly cocktail. Sorry, I just refuse to give it up. So, I gave up grains at dinnertime and now eat huge plate-fuls (I mean seriously huge, sometimes taking up the entire plate) of zero-point veggies and protein (shrimp, chicken, hamburger patty, whatever), just so I can have my predinner four-point cocktail. At the meeting today, I learned that I've lost 5 pounds in three weeks. Who says drinking can't work on a weight-loss plan?!"

A glass of wine several times a week is fine. But if you drink more like two glasses a day or you drink your week's quota over the weekend, then you need to take a hard look at how this little vice is influencing your mood, weight and health.

Moderation is the key, as is the size of that drink. The official "one drink" a day is 5 ounces of wine. The health benefits of wine or other alcoholic beverages also come from when, as well as how much, you drink. Wine goes from a health drink to a health problem after any more than six drinks a week for women. That is six drinks spread over six days, not gulped all at once during Friday night's happy hour. You can't drink your week's allotment of wine on Saturday and get the same health benefits as you would from one drink consumed daily. Besides, chug a bottle of Merlot and you've downed 500 to 600 calories, that's the equivalent of two Big Macs!

Just as you should eat slowly and mindfully, you also should develop the habit of drinking slowly. It takes the liver one to two hours to detoxify the alcohol in one drink. Drink any faster than that and alcohol accumulates in the blood and tissues. The buzz you feel means you are saturating your brain and tissues with the toxic effects of alcohol—you now have passed the point of reaping any of the health benefits of wine. Instead, follow the drinking rules laid out in Chapter 8.

Mmmmmm, Chocolate!

I'm a lifelong, hard-core chocoholic. I cannot think of a time when the sight or aroma of chocolate didn't leave my knees weak. My dad turned me onto rocky road candy in the early years, followed by my sister's divine chocolate chip cookies in my teens. While living in the dorms my freshman year of college, I polished off a 5-pound box of See's candy in a record three days.

You can imagine my relief when studies in the 1990s from the University of California at Davis, Harvard, and other respectable institutions found that chocolate isn't just a mood booster, an excuse to celebrate, a treat and a melt-in-your-mouth moment of ecstasy, it also is a powerhouse of antioxidants with the potential to lower heart disease, blood pressure and possibly cancer and diabetes. And get this one—it might even help you look younger and think faster! I was so thrilled to hear the news, I went right to the cupboard and celebrated with a Dove bar.

Our ancient ancestors would hardly be surprised at these findings, since chocolate originated hundreds of years ago as a medicinal plant. Chocolate's botanical name is *Theobroma cacao*, which roughly translates to "food of the gods." That title comes not just because chocolate has an incredibly pleasurable taste, but also because it was used first by the Aztecs and then later in Europe to treat hundreds of ailments from apathy and poor digestion to fertility and sexual prowess. (Casanova is said to have chosen chocolate over champagne as his aphrodisiac of choice, and Montezuma's household devoured 2,000 jars of chocolate a day!)

Of course, not all chocolate is created equal. Some is literally packed with health-enhancing antioxidants while other kinds are just packages of fat and sugar.

Getting to Know Chocolate

Chocolate comes from cacao beans, which are roasted, fermented and then crushed into a liquid called chocolate liquor. This liquor is pressed to separate out the fat (cocoa butter), leaving a cocoa "cake" or solid that is ground into cocoa powder. This powder contains powerful antioxidants, flavonoids such as procyanidins, epicatechins and catechins. These are the same compounds found in green tea and red wine that deactivate the cell-damaging oxygen fragments called free radicals.

Cocoa powder outranks just about any food studied when it comes to these antioxidants. The level of antioxidants can be measured in any food by a test called Oxygen Radical Absorption Capacity (ORAC). According to Ronald Prior, Ph.D., at the U.S. Department of Agriculture Arkansas Children's Nutrition Center, "A serving of dark chocolate measures 9,000 units on the ORAC scale, compared to an average of about 2,000 units found in typical servings of fruits or vegetables." That explains why a study from the University of Scranton found that chocolate contained more flavonoids than 23 different vegetables and several fruits. Other studies note that some chocolate has four times the level of catechins than does black tea. It is these phytonutrients that raise chocolate from pure pleasure to health protector. (See Chapter 5 for more about ORAC.)

Chocolate for Your Heart

As chocolate intake goes up, heart disease risk goes down. People who consume chocolate on a regular basis have almost a 20% lower risk for heart disease. The flavonoids in chocolate act much like aspirin to thin the blood and reduce the risk for deadly clots. They reduce inflammation of the artery walls associated with atherosclerosis and protect LDLs, the bad cholesterol, from being damaged by free radicals, which would make them sticky and more apt to clog arteries. Chocolate eaters also have higher levels of the good cholesterol, the HDLs. In short, feed people chocolate and their blood levels of antioxidants rise, their arteries become more elastic, their blood clots dissolve and their risk for heart disease drops. Just two weeks of including a snack-size chocolate bar (think Halloween candy) in the daily diet is enough to note improvements in antioxidant levels and artery function.

Chocolate also lowers blood pressure. The flavonoids in cocoa have a relaxing effect on blood vessels, likely because they increase the production of nitric oxide, which dilates arteries. As a result, blood vessels are more elastic and efficient at regulating blood pressure. Which explains why the more chocolate people consume, the lower their blood pressure. In fact, chocolate lovers have a 50% lower risk for dying from heart disease and a 47% lower risk for dying prematurely from any cause compared to chocolate abstainers.

Eat Chocolate: Look and Think Younger

The antioxidants in chocolate also might help you look younger, since they protect the skin from the damaging effects of sunshine. One study found that women who consumed drinks containing cocoa powder every day for three months had increased blood flow to the skin and 25% less sun damage associated with premature wrinkling, sunburn and skin cancer. The flavonols in cocoa increase blood flow to the brain, too. This might help send extra oxygen to brain tissue, which would improve mental performance.

A 5-Pound Box of Candy?

I have not set the best example with some of my past chocolate transgressions, like that 5-pound box of candy in the dorms. Granted, studies have found that the more cocoa powder people eat, the lower their disease risk. But there is a limit, typically set at about 1 ounce of dark chocolate several times a week.

"Chocolate can certainly be included in a healthy diet, but I wouldn't call it a health food," says Jeffrey Blumberg, Ph.D., Director of the Antioxidants Research Laboratory at the USDA Human Nutrition Research Center on Aging at Tufts University in Boston. A dark chocolate bar has the same amount of antioxidants as a cup of green tea, but the tea is calorie-free while the chocolate has more than 200 calories. Nibble one of those 3.5-ounce chocolate bars hawked at movie theaters and you've downed more than 500 calories.

The health benefits of chocolate begin to pale when compared to the wealth of vitamins, minerals, fiber, phytonutrients and more you get in broccoli, blueberries and other super mood foods. Besides, you won't control diabetes, heart disease or hypertension if you're packing on the pounds. That 5-pound box of chocolate I devoured totaled 11,520 calories. It took me a month to lose the more than 3 pounds I gained in those three days. No single food is the cause of the obesity epidemic, but anything that is as calorie-dense and delicious as chocolate is easy to overconsume.

Shopping Tips

Not everything chocolate deserves applause. In fact, many cheap chocolate candies have little or no health-redeeming benefits.

Steer clear of the chocolate creams: that's not cocoa butter inside those cream-filled centers, it is artery-clogging cream. The same goes for chocolate ice cream. Milk chocolate is a waste of time, at least in terms of the health and antioxidant value. On the other hand, the more cocoa powder in a chocolate bar, the higher the antioxidants and the better for you. No cocoa powder, no antioxidants.

Chocolate bars don't always list the antioxidant or cocoa content, so how do you know which bar to choose? In general, the darker the bar, the more cocoa. The one exception: the alkalizing salts used in Dutch-processed cocoa destroy flavonoids, cutting the total to half the original amount. In all other chocolates made from cocoa, the flavonoid content from highest to lowest, according to a recent study from Cornell University, is: cocoa powder, bittersweet baking chocolate, then dark chocolate, followed by baking chips. Milk chocolate contains about one-tenth the flavonoids of cocoa powder, since the cocoa has been diluted with sugar and milk. White chocolate, which contains no cocoa, has none.

When a bar does list the cocoa powder, choose products with at least 60% cocoa content, preferably 70% or more. Brands to look for include Lindt, El Rey, Scharffen Berger, Lake Champlain and Ghirardelli. Any chocolate bar with "Cocoapro" on the label also contains antioxidants, since these products use a patented process that protects the flavonoid content from being destroyed during processing.

How do you limit intake to a healthy serving of 1 to 2 ounces a few times a week without overindulging?

- Include a small amount of high-quality dark chocolate with meals or soon after. You're less likely to binge that way.
- Buy individually wrapped pieces, so it's portioned for you ahead of time.
- Use cocoa powder as the base of your chocolate treats, since it has no cocoa butter and is low in calories, yet packed with antioxidants.

Every chocoholic knows that abstinence does not work. Nothing satisfies a chocolate craving except chocolate. Plan guilt-free little indulgences throughout the week, and revel in all the good you are doing for your heart and health.

The Ultimate Cure for Cravings

Cravings might be hardwired into our brains, but that doesn't mean they are set in concrete. I can't tell you how many times over the years I have had people tell me they were totally powerless to a craving, yet found by making a few other changes in their diets that those cravings miraculously vanished.

Susan was a participant in one of my classes years ago when I was doing research for my book *The Origin Diet.* She confessed to me at the start of the program that she would try to follow my diet guidelines, but she had to have her can of cola every afternoon. It was a vice she refused to give up. I told her that was fine, just to follow the diet guidelines as closely as possible. By the second week of being on the diet, Susan was amazed to find she no longer needed her daily soda pop: "I can't believe that I only had one cola this week, and I didn't even really think about it. My other cravings, like for cheese, are pretty much gone, too!"

Natalie, another participant in one of my classes, was addicted to chocolate. But after following my advice to eat a small, nutritious breakfast and to bring healthful snacks with her every day, she found she no longer needed the chocolate. Natalie decided to keep chocolate in her weekly plan, even though the cravings had stopped. "Now I have a little piece sometimes, not because I have to, but because I want to," she says. "It's a big difference and I feel so much more in control."

SECRET 10:
EAT RIGHT AT NIGHT

The Promise

In two weeks of making this change, you will:

- notice an improvement in sleep patterns
- feel more rested during the day

In one month, you will:

- be more energized, with more even energy during the day
- sleep more soundly throughout the night
- feel less stressed
- think more clearly
- learn new tasks more easily
- remember more
- be less likely to binge on junk food

In one year, you will:

- lose up to 26 pounds

Bonnie is an accountant and mother of two small children in Phoenix. For years, she battled sleep problems. She had no trouble falling asleep, but several times a week she would wake at about 2:00 a.m. "My mind would start racing and I just couldn't get back to sleep," she says. "The most ridiculous worries and frets would pop into my head, thoughts I'd never entertain in the daytime. My heart would pound and it took me sometimes up to two hours to get back to sleep." The lack of sleep left her gritting her teeth, drinking coffee and nibbling sugary snacks all day to stay alert. At night she collapsed into bed and slept poorly, and the cycle would repeat itself.

I met Bonnie on a plane. We chatted from Phoenix to Minneapolis. When she learned I was a dietitian, she bombarded me with questions, oddly enough not about her sleep, but about how to lose the 45 pounds she'd gained during the past three years. She had no idea that the solution to her expanding waistline was in the bedroom as much as it was at the dinner table. By the time we landed in Minneapolis, she had a plan that would help solve both her insomnia and her weight problem.

Desperately Seeking Sleep

How well you sleep has a huge impact on your mood, energy level and weight. It is during sleep that your body repairs itself, stores energy for the next day, strengthens the immune system so you can successfully fight off infection and disease, and de-stresses, both mentally and physically.

During the deepest sleep, your body makes more of a hormone called HGH, or human growth hormone (HGH), that promotes growth and repair of all tissues, especially muscles. When you sleep poorly, your body makes less HGH, which means your muscles begin to break down. Lose muscle and your metabolism slows. Consequently, lack of sleep can lead to weight gain. It's a vicious cycle you don't want to enter, since once you gain weight, you are more likely to sleep poorly, which promotes weight gain, which promotes sleep problems, and you spiral into a big, fat problem.

Deep sleep also is the body's chance to lower stress hormone levels. Fail to get enough sleep, or sleep fitfully with frequent awakenings, and you cram those hormones into high gear, which speeds the aging process and increases the risk for a whole host of ills, from heart disease to diabetes. In fact, those who have trouble falling or staying asleep are more likely to die prematurely from any cause compared to well-rested people.

Ask any happy, fit person, and they will tell you that lack of sleep also is a big, fat no-no if you want to be upbeat, smart or energized. Since sleep is where your brain sorts, consolidates, processes and stores the ton of information gathered and downloaded during the day, it is obvious how important a good night's sleep is for learning, thinking, remembering and being creative. People who sleep well show a 44% improvement in memory compared to less-rested people.

The worse you feel, the more likely you'll eat—and all the wrong stuff, since fatigue and the blues dissolve your resolve to take care of yourself. The walking dead are in survival mode with the attitude that "I'll eat whatever it takes to feel better right now."

Combine the lack of HGH with the extra calories sleep-deprived people eat in a misguided attempt to stay alert, and it's no wonder this scenario leads to weight gain. On the other hand, you literally can sleep your way thin, just like Janice did: "I used to overeat and eat all the wrong stuff. Then I figured out that my hectic schedule and lack of sleep was to blame. As long as I stay well rested, I notice my cravings for carbs drop, but when I'm tired I really want them. A good night's sleep was all I needed to ignore the temptation." Sleep-deprived people, like Janice and Bonnie, who finally start sleeping well lose about half a pound of body fat a week, which equates to a 26-pound loss of fat in one year. Bonnie lost more than that, but that's because she had a few issues at the dinner table to correct, too.

Lack of sleep → ↑ stress hormones +
↓ HGH → ↑ appetite, ↑ fat storage,
↑ weight gain, and ↓ muscle and ↓ memory

Are You Chasing Mr. Sandman?

- Are you sleep deprived?
- How much sleep do you really need?

Those questions depend entirely on the unique person that is you. It's a no-brainer you are probably sleep deprived if you can't fall asleep, log less than six hours of sleep a night or wake up too early and can't get back to sleep. On the other hand, you are probably getting enough sleep if you wake refreshed and ready to go, feel energized throughout the day and fall asleep at night within 20 minutes. The middle ground—that zone between exuberance and coma—is more difficult to decipher.

Where you are on the sleep scale might be more clear if you ask yourself a few questions. If you answer "yes, that's me" to three or more of the following statements, consider yourself a card-carrying member of the snooze-deprived set.

1. Getting up in the morning is one tough job. I absolutely need an alarm clock, but even then I sometimes hit the snooze button and fall back to sleep.

2. I can't make it through the morning and afternoon without caffeinated beverages, like coffee, tea, colas or energy drinks.

3. I am easily irritated by minor upsets and sometimes snap at family, friends or coworkers only because I am tired.

4. I am groggy enough that I have trouble concentrating on tasks throughout the day.

5. I frequently have major waves of drowsiness at work or school or even while I'm driving.

6. I used to have hobbies or activities I loved to do, but I'm just too tired to participate anymore.

7. I feel old, worn-out, and like I have somehow lost my pizzazz.

8. I catch colds and flu more easily than in the past. I've had at least two bouts of some kind of illness or cold in the past six months.

9. Alcohol hits me harder than it used to.

10. I fall asleep within five minutes of my head hitting the pillow.

If you know sleep is a problem but you can't figure out why, it might help to keep a sleep journal for two weeks. Keeping a log of what happened during the day, along with your eating habits, can help you identify when and how you snooze and how activities, events, your diet or drinking habits and stress are affecting sleep.

This worked for me last year when all of a sudden I started waking up in the middle of the night with my heart racing. The sleep journal clearly showed that eating salty foods in the evening was triggering heart palpitations in the middle of the night. I'd never been salt sensitive before, but apparently my chemistry had changed. I've stopped eating anything salty after 7:00 p.m., and I make sure to drink lots of water and decaf tea to flush out any extra salt. As a result, I'm back to sleeping soundly all night.

Eat to Sleep

If you toss and turn, wake too early or have trouble falling asleep, your problem might be not in the bedroom but at the table. Granted, many of life's little challenges can upset a good night's sleep, including stress, depression, jet lag, hot flashes during menopause, a snoring partner or even the glow from your alarm clock. But what and how much you eat and drink from midday to bedtime has a huge effect on how well you sleep at night.

Your Sleep Log

Make copies of this sheet and use it every day for two weeks. Look for patterns that provide insight into why you sleep some nights and not others. Also, check out Peter Hauri and Shirley Linde's book, *No More Sleepless Nights,* for more detailed information on how to keep and analyze a sleep journal.

During the day	
1. Caffeine intake (how much and when)	
2. Alcohol intake (how much and when)	
3. Medications taken	
4. Dinner: spicy, gassy, big, fatty?	
5. Evening snack	
6. Overall day's diet (excellent, good, bad)	
7. How many minutes of vigorous exercise?	
8. Stress level (high, medium, low)	
9. What caused you stress today?	
10. Energy level (energetic, tired)	
11. Worry level (high, moderate, low)	
12. Joy level (high, moderate, low)	
13. Laughter (often, seldom, never)	
14. Did you nap? If so, how long and when	
At night	
15. Did you take anything to help you sleep?	
16. What time did you go to bed?	
17. How long did it take to fall asleep?	
18. Did you wake up during sleep? If so, how often and for how long?	
19. Thoughts while awake in the middle of the night	
20. What do you do when you wake up in the middle of the night?	
21. Wake-up time in the morning	
22. Compared to typical sleep, how would you rate last night's slumber?	
23. How refreshed and alert were you when you got up this morning?	

Date

Mon.	Tues.	Wed.	Thurs.	Fri.	Sat.	Sun.

The Natural High

Eat a light evening meal, cut back on sleep disturbers like caffeine and have a light all-carb snack at night to boost brain levels of serotonin and you will work with your body's natural rhythm and chemistry to help you sleep like a baby.

Caffeine: Roadblock to Dreamland

Let's start with midafternoon. As mentioned in Chapter 8, drinking coffee or any caffeinated beverage after about noon could be a big mistake. Caffeine revs the nervous system and lowers levels of a sleep hormone called melatonin. If you are one of the people sensitive to this little drug, then it could linger in your system for up to 12 hours.

Many people are totally oblivious to how caffeine affects them. A member of my family swears coffee has no effect on her. She drinks it right up until she goes to bed at night. Yet the next morning (over coffee) she will tell anyone who will listen all about the problems people around the country are having with their spouses, children, friends and family. How does she know this? Is she psychic? Is she tuning into some cosmic pool of Dr. Phil rejects? Nope. She's been up all night listening to talk radio shows! But caffeine doesn't affect her at all, or so she says!

The Experiment

If you struggle with sleep problems, you might try a little caffeine experiment: eliminate all caffeine from your diet for two weeks. It will take a few days for the withdrawal headaches to subside and for the caffeine to drain from your system. After that, pay attention to your sleep habits. Do they improve? If so, you know caffeine was tinkering with your doze control. You can probably drink coffee or tea in the morning, but definitely steer clear of the stuff after noon.

Besides the beverages, don't eat chocolate or take any over-the-counter medications (OTCs) that contain caffeine during your two-week experiment. A 6-ounce cup of regular coffee contains about 85 milligrams of caffeine. That's nothing compared to two Extra-Strength Excedrin tablets. Take those and you've just swallowed 130 milligrams of caffeine, which is close to the caffeine in a Monster Energy or Full Throttle drink! In one study of 3,000 men and women, those who took caffeine-containing medications were twice as likely to have trouble falling asleep as those who took the same medication without caffeine.

Before purchasing any OTC drug, read the label under "active ingredients," where you'll find mention of caffeine. Other medications that might rev you up or keep you from catching your quota of *zzzs* include phenylpropanolamine in some cold medications, thyroid medications and diuretic medications (take them in the evening and you might be up half the night with jaunts to the bathroom). Even a stick of Jolt Caffeinated gum, coffee yogurt and coffee-flavored ice cream has enough caffeine to keep you tossing and turning. Cut them out during your two-week experiment and see if you sleep better.

The Evening Train to Snoozeville

Happy, fit people know that what they choose to eat at dinner can make or break their sleep habits. This was where Bonnie had tripped up on her chances for rest. Her biggest meal of the day was dinner, and her favorite foods were spicy Mexican fare, such as enchiladas seasoned with chili peppers and salsa. The jar of Tums by her bedside was a red flag that something other than stress was the cause of her night awakenings.

Evenings can be the most challenging time when it comes to snacking, overeating and munching on all the wrong stuff.

Feast or Famine?

Have you ever pushed back from the Thanksgiving feast, staggered to the living room, collapsed in the recliner and nodded off? If you can relate to food coma, then you know that a great big meal in the evening makes most people groggy. But just because you fall asleep doesn't mean you sleep soundly. In fact, big or fatty meals might put you out at first, but they actually keep you from sleeping soundly through the night.

It takes hours to thoroughly digest a great big meal. Like a washing machine on the large-load cycle, your stomach and intestines will be churning for at least four hours, maybe more, after a big greasy meal. An overactive digestive tract revs metabolism and keeps the body "active" for hours. With your body's factory of organs, tissues and cells in full production, it's difficult to completely relax into a deep sleep. Sure, you are groggy, but that's because blood has been diverted from your brain to your digestive tract to handle the glut of food and fat. Basically, you are oxygen deprived, and that makes you sleepy.

In addition, a large wad of food in your stomach can press against the little trapdoor that separates your stomach from your esophagus (the tube that runs from your throat to your stomach). The pressure can cause food, along with stomach acid, to trickle up, leading to heartburn, acid reflux and even gastroesophageal reflux disease (GERD). On the other hand, keep the evening meal light and low-fat and eat no less than three hours before bedtime, and you stack the deck in favor of sleeping like a baby all night.

Keep dinner light—approximately 500 to 700 calories—and focus on quick-digesting super mood foods, such as vegetables, salads, fruit, whole grains and low-fat milk or soy milk. Complement this plate with small amounts of extra-lean meat, poultry breast or omega-rich fish, such as salmon. The protein in the meat or seafood (or milk, legumes and low-fat cheese) will help keep you satisfied and less likely to nibble at the refrigerator later in the evening or in the middle of the night.

The Natural High

Exercise every day and you will fall asleep faster, sleep deeper, and sleep longer than if you were a couch potato.

Two Weeks of Light and Healthy Super Mood Food Dinners

The evening meal should be light and low-fat. It also is a great time to pack in some of those super mood foods discussed in Chapter 5. Pay close attention to portions, since even superfoods can pack on the pounds and disrupt sleep if consumed in excess. Here is two weeks' worth of supper ideas:

1. Grilled salmon, asparagus, whole-grain couscous and a tossed spinach salad with low-fat dressing.

2. Grilled halibut, sweet potato fries, Mango Craisins, Avocado Toss* and tomato juice.

3. Small grilled flank steak served with mashed potatoes (made with fat-free half & half and whipped with chopped spinach or chard), Orange-glazed Roasted Brussels Sprouts and Cauliflower* and a glass of calcium-fortified orange juice.

4. Spinach and Roasted Red Pepper Frittata* served with whole-wheat bread, orange slices and tossed salad. For dessert, dried tart cherries mixed into yogurt.

5. Small piece of grilled pork tenderloin, Cherry- & Apple-Stuffed Acorn Squash*, carrots and a glass of low-fat milk or soy milk.

6. Linguini à la Pomodori*, mixed vegetables and low-fat milk or soy milk. For dessert, Spiced Panna Cotta with Strawberry-Shiraz Compote*.

7. Roast turkey breast, zucchini sauteed in chicken broth and herbs, Mashed Roasted Sweet Potatoes with a Taste of Honey* and 3-bean salad. For dessert, diced kiwi mixed into yogurt.

8. Fish tacos made with corn tortillas, grilled halibut, shredded cabbage, diced tomatoes, diced avocado and fat-free sour cream. Serve with sweet potato fries, steamed vegetables and sparkling water with lemon.

9. Grilled shrimp and vegetable kabobs over brown rice. Serve with steamed Chinese pea pods. For dessert, a glass of Orange Cranberry Fizz*.

10. Small slice meatloaf, peas and carrots, roasted red potatoes and a spinach salad with low-fat dressing.

11. Sage-Infused Roasted Butternut Squash Soup*, whole-wheat bread and a tossed salad with mandarin oranges and low-fat dressing.

12. Chicken burritos made with tortillas with DHA filled with chicken breast, corn, spinach leaves, black beans (optional), red pepper slices and salsa (optional). Serve with apple and orange slices topped with yogurt and a glass of tomato juice.

13. Curried Butternut Squash with Chutney and Rice*, tomato slices and low-fat milk or soy milk. For dessert, grapes, orange slices and kiwi sprinkled with cashews.

14. A big bowl of romaine lettuce topped with grilled chicken slices, corn, red onion slices (optional), red pepper slices and low-fat dressing. Serve with a slice of sourdough bread. For dessert, Vanilla Cream Sprinkled with Nuts*.

* See Recipes section.

De-spice It Up

Bonnie loved spicy food. But it didn't love her. That big, spicy meal toward the end of the day wreaked havoc with her stomach in the middle of the night. The heartburn woke her up, and once she was awake, her worries took over and kept her tossing for hours. She took my advice and cut back on the size and spiciness of her evening meals and within weeks she had put the Tums away and was sleeping soundly through the night.

Heartburn. Indigestion. Bloating. Gas. None of these are welcome bedfellows. Yet your choices at dinner could be the very reason they invade the bedroom late at night. If stomach upsets keep you up at night, here are the four habits to cease and desist immediately:

- Douse your dinner meal with chilies, garlic, red pepper flakes, Tabasco or even spaghetti sauce or cucumbers for those with tender tummies and you may be up at 2:00 a.m. rummaging through the cabinets looking for an antacid.

- Monosodium glutamate or MSG might enhance the flavor of your favorite foods, but it also can disrupt sleep and cause vivid nightmares and restlessness. Check labels and ask waiters when dining out to guarantee you avoid any food made with this additive.

- Gas-forming foods, from super mood foods like beans, broccoli, lentils and peppers to Brussels sprouts, cabbage, cucumbers and radishes can puff you up with gas like a helium balloon, which interferes with a sound sleep.

- Wolf your food and you swallow air along with the barely chewed meal. That combination leads to bloating, gas and cramping in the middle of the night as the food and air make it into your intestines.

The Nightcap

Alcohol is the most common sleep aid for insomniacs. But what people think helps them to sleep could be the very thing that leaves them sleep deprived.

A glass of wine or hot toddy in the evening might make you sleepy, but drink too much and alcohol interferes with a good night's sleep. Alcohol helps you fall asleep and might even help you sleep soundly for the first hour or so. After that, it disrupts the rapid eye movement sleep (REM), which is the sleep phase where you dream and release the day's tensions. Alcohol also leads to more night awakenings, more restless sleep and less of your sleeping time spent in deep sleep, called delta sleep.

Another problem with using alcohol as your sleep partner is that it is easy to build up a tolerance. While a glass of wine helped relax you and got you to sleep last year, keep it up and pretty soon it takes two or three glasses to get the same effect. Women are especially vulnerable to this cycle, since their smaller body size and slower metabolism of alcohol means they get a bigger alcohol punch from the same number of drinks compared to men. People who notice that they sleep less soundly or wake up more frequently on the nights when they drink socially should avoid alcohol altogether before bedtime.

Alcohol at night also could make you stupid the next day. Memories are created by strengthening connections between groups of brain cells. Much of this work happens while you sleep, with brain cells tinkering with those networks, increasing some and reducing others during that REM phase of sleep. As a result, you don't learn or process information as well when you drink. This might explain why people who learn a new skill then have an alcoholic beverage before they go to sleep lose about 40% of the knowledge and perform much worse the next day compared to people who skipped the nightcap.

In short, a glass of wine with dinner is fine, but don't overdo it. Definitely steer clear of alcohol if you notice from your sleep log that it leaves you short on shut-eye.

Bedtime Snacks

Want to sleep like a baby? You are most likely to do that when your levels of the brain chemical serotonin are high. As discussed in Chapter 3, serotonin is made from an amino acid called tryptophan. The more tryptophan in the brain, the more serotonin is made and the better you sleep.

There is a perfectly safe, natural way to raise tryptophan levels: a handful of carbs about an hour before you turn off the light. "A light snack of carbohydrate-rich foods, say crackers and fruit or popcorn, just before bedtime probably won't have much of an effect on how fast a person falls asleep, but it may help some people sleep longer and more soundly," says Gary Zammit, Ph.D., Director of the Sleep Disorders Institute at St. Luke's Hospital in New York City.

But don't overdo it. It only takes about 30 grams of carbs to get the serotonin effect. Any more than that and you're just adding unwanted calories and possibly interfering with sleep by stuffing too much food into your stomach.

Some people swear a warm glass of milk puts a hefty dose of *zzzs* into their slumber. It's not because of the tryptophan in milk, which is a building block for serotonin, since the protein in milk will block tryptophan getting into the brain (see page 183 for more on tryptophan and serotonin). It must be that the soothing, warm liquid raises body temperature a degree or two, which relaxes the body and signals that it is bedtime.

Evening Craving Control

If you have a hard time putting a lid on evening nibbling, you might need to set some ground rules. For example, the biggest obstacle to weight loss for Jill, a waitress in San Diego, was her nighttime eating: "I would get home from work, tired and in need of some comfort. I'd eat a great dinner, but then would want something sweet. I'd end up nibbling all night on whatever was in the cupboard or fridge." When I tallied Jill's calorie intake in evening snacks, she was shocked to learn she was gobbling more than 1,500 calories before bedtime.

If you are like Jill, you might want to make a rule that there is no eating in bed, no eating while watching TV or maybe no food two hours before bedtime. Or perhaps you decide to not bring temptation into the house at all or to have the kids clean the kitchen after dinner, so you don't have to venture near food after the evening meal. Just remember, failure to plan is planning to fail. Make those rules and stick with them!

Super Mood Foods for Sleep

Follow the real-foods diet guidelines in this book and you should notice improvements in sleep, along with mood, energy and brain power. That's because you'll be getting all the vitamins, minerals, fiber, phytonutrients and quality carbs in the right balance to aid in optimal energy throughout the day and maximum sleep power at night. What a difference compared to fueling your body on junk!

Well-nourished people are happier, leaner, healthier and sleep better. It just makes sense. Like a fine-tuned machine, your body runs and rests best when supplied with the right mix of the right fuel at the right time. For example,

- **Legumes and wheat germ:** These foods supply ample B vitamins, like folic acid and vitamins B_6 and B_{12}, which are assembly-line workers in the production of serotonin and sleep. Boost intake of these vitamins and insomniacs report improvements in sleep within a few weeks.

- **Milk, yogurt and soy milk:** These foods are rich in calcium and magnesium, two minerals essential for muscle relaxation and nerve transmission. Magnesium also plays a key role in body chemistry that regulates sleep. Deficiencies of either one can cause muscle cramps, increased stress and poor sleep, while optimal intake decreases the time it takes to fall asleep, increases deep sleep and improves brain waves during sleep.

- **Dark green leafy vegetables and legumes:** These foods supply iron, which helps lower the risk for restless leg syndrome, an uncomfortable burning, itching or tickling sensation in the legs, arms or torso that disrupts sleep.

- **Fatty fish or DHA-fortified foods:** These healthy fats improve sleep patterns, possibly because they help boost melatonin, the hormone that regulates the sleep and wake cycle. Even babies sleep better and longer when their mothers consumed optimal levels of DHA during pregnancy.

Dose to Doze

What if there was a pill that could solve all your sleep problems? While nothing works as well as eating right and taking care of yourself, there are a few options in the pill department that you might want to ponder.

Melatonin

Melatonin is a hormone made naturally in the body and released at night or in the dark. It helps regulate the cycle of waking and sleeping. Some people don't make enough, especially as they get older, which leaves them tossing and turning.

Can you compensate for low levels by taking a supplement of melatonin? Maybe. Studies show a slight improvement in sleep, especially in speed of falling asleep, when people take melatonin supplements. Melatonin also helps curb the nasty sleep-deprivation associated with jet lag. It's not as clear whether melatonin helps keep people asleep, if it increases the deep sleep that people need the most, or even if they feel more rested when taking melatonin for sleep problems.

How much should you take? If you decide to give melatonin a try, a short-term daily dose of between 0.5 and 5 milligrams appears to be safe. Take these supplements close to bedtime or at the expected bedtime at your destination when you are traveling across several time zones.

Most melatonin supplements are made from a synthetic form of the hormone and are available in liquid, tablet and intranasal sprays. They come in immediate-release and extended-release formulas. Since a short-lived, high-peak dose of melatonin is most effective, it is probably best to use an immediate-release product. The extended release forms of the supplement don't work as well.

One last word of caution: most experts caution against taking melatonin supplements for any longer than a month. Short-term use appears safe, but the lack of long-term studies has left safety issues hanging. In addition, make sure to take those supplements in the evening, since taking too much melatonin at the wrong time may worsen sleep problems.

Valerian

Valerian is an herbal remedy for sleep problems used as far back as Ancient Greece. The root and stems are used to make a tea or tincture, or you can take tablets or capsules of the dried herb.

Valerian appears to work. In one study, people took 400 milligrams of a valerian extract or placebos. Those who took valerian fell asleep faster, slept better and had fewer night awakenings. Studies have compared valerian to sleeping pills and found they both worked, but the valerian had fewer side effects. Other studies, however, have found no benefits to taking valerian, so more research is needed.

No one knows just how valerian works, or even what an optimal dose is. A typical dose for short-term use ranges from 400 to 900 milligrams. Many compounds isolated in the herb have been suspected, but it is more likely that it is a combination of ingredients, rather than just one or two, that is doing the job. The good news is that no harmful side effects have been noted. To be on the safe side, pregnant women, people on other sedatives and young children should not take this herb.

5-HTP

In the days when tryptophan supplements were available, studies showed that popping a tryptophan pill decreased the time it took to fall asleep by up to 50% and improved the soundness and length of sleep. Since you can't get tryptophan pills any more (they were banned back in the 1980s because of a serious contamination problem), companies now make a replacement, 5-hydroxy-L-tryptophan or 5-HTP. The

body makes 5-HTP from tryptophan, and like tryptophan, 5-HTP is converted to serotonin in the brain.

Supplements of 5-HTP show promise in helping
with insomnia, weight loss and even panic attacks.
Numerous studies show people sleep better and
longer when they take 5-HTP. Safety issues linger,
however, and no one is quite sure about the best
dose (as little as 20 to as much as 300 milligrams for
adults has been used) or the consequences of taking
5-HTP for months and years. Enteric-coated tablets are
recommended to increase absorption and minimize
potential side effects, such as stomach discomfort,
nausea and vomiting. The less you take, the less
likely you'll suffer side effects. If you are considering
taking 5-HTP, consult your physician first, especially
if you are pregnant or breast-feeding, have high blood
pressure or diabetes or take mood-altering medications
or herbs.

Move to Snooze

You knew it was coming. I can't in all good conscience
fail to mention how important daily exercise is to
nighttime sleeping. Happy, fit people exercise almost
every day, which in part explains why they sleep so
soundly. Exercise for at least 45 minutes any time of
the day except just before you go to bed, and it will
help burn stress hormones, so you aren't left stewing
in your own juices all night long. Exercisers get a third

more deep sleep than couch potatoes, while crabby people who take up exercise fall asleep faster, sleep deeper and sleep longer than they did before they started moving.

Exercise has been the ticket to dreamland for many of my friends and clients, such as Janice:

"I sleep much better on days I run than on days I don't. I even ran through the seventh month with both pregnancies. When both the kids were little, I ran with them in a double jogger-stroller. The kids have my number! When I haven't run in a few days, I get cranky, and the kids will plead, 'Mom, please, go for a run!' They know!"

As another client, Julie, puts it, "Exercise allows me to concentrate more, sleep better and think more clearly. End of story."

Sleep Yourself Happy

Seeking *zzz*s might be as simple as making a few changes in when, what and how much you eat. In addition, adopt a relaxing bedtime routine that helps prepare you for sleep, like taking a hot bath or reading a book. For serious and chronic problems, always consult your physician.

SECRET 11:
THE ONE HABIT YOU MUST EMBRACE TO BE HAPPY, FIT AND HEALTHY

The Promise

In one hour of making this change, you will:

- be happier, calmer and more confident
- have more energy
- see an improvement in your day

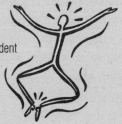

In one month, you will:

- be less stressed
- sleep better
- experience less fatigue
- have a more even, upbeat attitude

In one year, you will:

- notice an improvement in memory
- lose lots of weight
- slow the aging process
- lower your risk for all age-related diseases
- look younger
- have more confidence, self-esteem and pride in yourself and your accomplishments
- increase your chances for moments of bliss

I have been blessed with several moments of bliss in my life. Some just descended on me like a heavenly warm blanket in times of need. A few came during my midtwenties, before kids and when I was disciplined enough to meditate every day. But most moments of sheer joy have come during and because of exercise.

The most profound "moment" of bliss lasted an entire week while I pedaled almost 300 miles through Glacier National Park in Montana and Canada. The terrain was glorious—rugged peaks dotted with mountain goats and curly-horned sheep—separated by green valleys, with vistas that would make anyone's knees weak from the grandeur. The ride was supported—all I had to do was bike, eat and sleep. It was the most vigorous physical exertion I had tackled in many years, with several days of pedaling uphill continuously for 5 miles or more, then doing that over and over, totaling 50 to 100 miles from early morning to late afternoon.

You might ask why I took on such a challenge. The short answer is "to see if I could do it." The longer answer has to do with being in my late fifties and figuring, if not now, when? The trip paid off in ways I never expected.

When I'd summited the Highway to the Sun on the second day, reaching the Continental Divide at 6,646 feet, something besides my sanity snapped. I entered a state of sheer joy that lasted the rest of the trip. At first, I was just ecstatic to have conquered the mountain, dancing about and high-fiving anyone who would put up their hand. That initial high was followed by a more lasting gratitude and appreciation. As I began the descent, everything seemed perfect, absolutely right with the world. There was nothing to fear; I had no anxiety, no worries. I was in a state of complete peace. I went to bed blissful and woke each morning after that knowing in my heart that the day would be perfect.

During that week, I often thought of my dad, who had been gone for almost 15 years. He loved nature and the outdoors. As I pedaled through Glacier, I knew he would have felt right at home with the valleys, rivers and mountains, and I wondered if he had ever been here. I thought about his later years, when he no longer could fly-fish on the Rogue River or walk in the mountains and instead we drove through the Carson Valley in Nevada playing a game of who could spot the most red-tailed hawks. He always won. I swear he could spot a hawk a mile away.

On the third day of the bike trip, as I pedaled alone along a flower-speckled valley, in a state of sheer gratitude and with my dad on my mind, a red-tailed hawk swooped down and flew eye level with me. It soared alongside my bike as I pedaled. Just me and that red-tailed hawk with the wind at our backs and the Rocky Mountain sunshine in our faces. That hawk never looked at me; he just flew alongside as I sailed down the road, as if to say, "I just came by to tell you that your dad says 'hello.'" After about a quarter of a mile, the hawk veered back off across the valley. It was the most amazing experience. In that state of grace, I was open to a sweet message from someone very dear to me.

Being physically active has given me a thousand and one moments of happiness, pride, gratitude, joy and bliss. But the day I flew with the red-tailed hawk topped them all. It was a blissful exclamation point on a glorious week of joy.

I can't promise exercise will always bring you moments of bliss, but I can promise that for every hour you invest in physical activity, your body will pay you back a hundredfold with better physical, emotional, mental and possibly even spiritual health. It also will jump-start your quality of life today and extend your young years far into the future (most of the folks I rode with on the Glacier ride were well past 50!). In fact, one aerobics class is enough to boost your mood. Hey, even a brisk 10-minute walk can help lift your spirits and soothe the edges of fatigue, anger, confusion or anxiety. It is the best investment you will ever make in your life and your health.

The Natural High

Our bodies were designed over millions of years to be vigorously active. It is not that exercise is "good" for us. It is that when we don't move that the system breaks down. Nothing you do will have as big an impact on your weight, mood and health both today and down the road as exercise.

Butt Exercises

Americans average almost 60% of the day sitting on their butts. We sit to eat, drive, watch television, work and play at computers and ride lawn mowers. We sit at movies, ball games, plays, concerts, meetings, coffee shops and restaurants. We sit in airports and airplanes, buses and trains, trucks and golf carts. Add all those hours of sitting with the seven to nine hours of sleeping, and it is easy to see there is not much time left for moving. Even if you plan a half-hour walk at lunchtime, that still leaves 23½ hours where your heart rate may not rise above an idle.

All that sitting means a fast trip to the fat farm! You burn next to no calories while sitting, or about 5 calories more an hour than you would if you were asleep. Do the math.

Excess sitting escalates the aging process. When our main occupation is sitting, we lose 1% to 2% of our muscle mass each year starting sometime in our thirties. That equates to a 5 to 10 pound loss of muscle every decade. As we lose muscle, which is the body's active tissue, our metabolism slows, so it is easy to pack on the pounds. As our metabolism slows, we become sluggish and tire easily and our moods plummet. The more we sit, the more fat accumulates around the middle, which escalates risks for all age-related diseases, from heart disease to dementia. Middle-age spread is the beginning of a continuum that if not stopped likely will end with living in a wheelchair or walker. It's not a pretty picture, and it doesn't have to happen.

Get Off Your "But"

Daily exercise is the fast track to weight loss and slowed aging. For example, Maureen, a freelance writer in the Pacific Northwest, made a few changes in her eating habits and kicked up the exercise to reach her weight goals: "I worked with a trainer once a week for the first six months and twice a week the second six months, doing strength training with bursts of cardio in between sets (like running up a short flight of stairs 10 times or jumping up on a raised step for one minute). The past two months, I added Pilates twice a week." That effort paid off. Maureen has lost 30 pounds so far and is still losing.

Exercise also has a domino effect on the rest of your habits, helping you eat better and take better care of yourself. That's what Victoria, a freelance writer and mother of two young children in Beaverton, Oregon, realized once she started moving more. "I learned as I got older that I must exercise to maintain my figure. No more 'buts' for me, like 'I should exercise, *but* I'm too busy.' Now I bike (either outside or on the stationary) every other day, lift weights a few times a week, and do Pilates a few times a week. Exercise naturally makes me want to eat healthier foods."

Staying lean doesn't just mean pumping iron or taking a spin class at the gym (although those are definitely good ideas, too). Often all a happy, fit person must do to avoid the bulge is keep moving during the day. Lean people use the stairs instead of the elevator, walk up the escalator rather than stand as if it were an amusement-park ride, and get up to turn the TV channel or talk to a coworker rather than use the remote or email. They move approximately two and a half hours more each day than their overweight buddies just by living actively, so they burn about 350 calories more. Over the course of a year, that could add up to as much as a 37-pound weight loss.

More important, everyone who maintains a significant amount of weight loss exercises. That's what researchers at Brown University found in their ongoing National Weight Control Registry study, where they have been following thousands of people who have maintained a significant weight loss for five years or more. More than 90% of them are moving every day for at least an hour to an hour and a half. Most of them walk, but many mix it up a bit, walking one day, swimming or taking an aerobics class the next day. Nothing you do will have as big an impact on your weight, as well as your mood and health both today and in the future, as exercise.

Use or Lose It

The older you get, the higher the stakes and the more important it is to get up and get moving.

I met Harold on a 70-mile bike ride through the Willamette Valley East of Salem, Oregon. When I asked him why he liked bicycling, he said, "I retired 10 years ago. I'd seen what happened to my coworkers and friends who retired. They sat in recliners and got stiff, cranky and old. I didn't want that to happen to me." So Harold dusted off an old three-speed he had in the garage and started to pedal around the neighborhood. That turned into an hour ride most evenings. "I crossed paths with the local bicycle club one night and decided it was time to kick it up a notch. I bought a better bike, joined the club, and here I am." Harold has lost 25 pounds since he retired, is medication free, runs circles around his other retired friends, and says, at 75 years young, "I've never been happier or more fit in my life."

Anyone who wants to age gracefully—with vigor, passion and independence—must exercise. That lesson came through loud and clear to me a few years back when I joined the gym. It was right after my mom had died and I had spent a good part of my time visiting her in the nursing home, where people in their seventies, eighties and beyond spent their time talking about who had died, who was sick and what aches and pains they were battling today.

In contrast, at the gym, I was surrounded by the same age group, but these people were from another planet. They were vigorous and enthusiastic. They flirted with each other and even with me. While they walked on the treadmills, pedaled the exercise cycles or lifted weights, they talked about what college courses they were taking or their next trip to India. Others, such as Helen, were battling diseases like cancer; it was exercise that kept them strong and their attitudes positive through treatment. Still others, like Roy, had at one time been on the verge of moving to an assisted living home: "I was riddled with aches and pains that I assumed were just part of aging. Turns out, once I started exercising, most of that pain went away. I guess I am a lot younger than I thought."

Not only does exercise keep heart and arteries squeaky clean and blood pressure low, it actually slows the aging process right at the very heart of our being—in the DNA or genes. Each strand of DNA in every cell in the body has handles at each end, much like the handles on a jump rope. Those handles are called telomeres. Their job is to keep the DNA from unraveling when it divides to make a new cell. The telomere handle shortens just a bit every time the cell divides. After many divisions, the cell's telomeres are so short they no longer protect the DNA, and the cell dies. The accumulation of dead cells is one marker for aging.

Anything that protects the telomeres from shortening prolongs the life of the cell, which in turn will prolong tissue health and prevent aging in general. Research shows that exercise protects telomeres from shortening. In fact, people who exercise at least three hours a week have much longer telomeres than couch potatoes, a difference that equates to slowing the aging process by 10 years!

A Few Reasons Why Everyone Should Exercise

Daily exercise:

- lowers the risk for heart disease, diabetes hypertension, cancer, stroke and almost all age-related diseases

- reduces the risk for depression and anxiety

- helps cope with stress

- elevates mood

- improves flexibility, strength and balance
- improves joint function and strengthens bones
- helps slim figures and burn body fat
- improves sleep
- raises energy levels and reduces fatigue
- enhances feelings of well-being
- improves appearance
- encourages better eating habits
- gives vitality a jump start
- boosts self-esteem, confidence and self-worth

The Number One Most Effective Antidepressant

If you are feeling down, are battling the winter blues or postpartum depression or are full-blown clinically depressed, exercise is the most effective treatment and cure. And it comes with no side effects and is free!

Thousands of studies spanning decades of research show over and over again that regular exercise is as effective as medication in boosting mood in most people, young and old, male and female. It helps people with mild to severe depression, people unresponsive to antidepressants, recovering alcoholics, people battling life-threatening illnesses such as cancer and people recovering from eating disorders. "Exercise relieves depression better than any antidepressant medication, counseling or even a combination of the two," says Ed Pierce, Ph.D., Associate Professor in the Department of Health and Sports Science at the University of Richmond.

What about people who are already happy? Julie, the public relations executive in Minneapolis, considers herself a happy person but loves the extra boost she gets from daily exercise: "Exercise definitely energizes me. My daily workout lets me concentrate more, sleep better and think more clearly. I don't feel myself without it."

Why Is Exercise So Good for Your Mood?

It's no surprise that exercise is Mother Nature's antidepressant, since it tweaks and adjusts a slew of brain chemicals, all in favor of a *natural high*. A daily workout raises levels of epinephrine and norepinephrine that enhance alertness. It increases serotonin levels, which brightens mood in much the same way as mood-elevating medications, such as Prozac. The rise in body temperature that results from a vigorous workout also has a tranquilizing effect on the body, not unlike soaking in a hot bath. Finally, the hour at the gym or the brisk walk is a break in the day's hectic schedule, a time-out from worries and unpleasant emotions.

Danielle, a coach and teacher in Salem, Oregon, uses exercise as her time to de-stress and problem solve:

"I am the type of person who worries about everything. Over the years I've learned to save my worry time for when I run. Exercise is such an invigorating experience that it allows my positive attitude to carry over into whatever I am thinking or worrying about. I'll run six miles and for the first two I have a lump in my throat and tears streaming down my face. But somewhere in the midst of that I can pick up the pace, push up a hill and let go of whatever is bothering me. By the end of the run, the problem doesn't feel so overwhelming, and I'm calmer, wiser and more at peace with myself and my life."

Danielle's jog-induced sanity could be caused by changes in brain chemistry, or perhaps it results from the notorious "runners' high," that feeling of euphoria following intense physical activity. This natural high has been attributed to endorphins, the body's natural morphinelike chemicals that help improve pain tolerance and generate feelings of euphoria and satisfaction.

Whatever the cause, one thing seems clear, and that is that exercise is a great natural antidepressant. Study after study supports the benefits of daily activity on mood. For example,

- Researchers at Stanford University compared the effects of no exercise with various intensities of exercise on psychological outcomes. After one year, the exercisers had significantly less stress, anxiety and depression compared to their sedentary counterparts, regardless of whether they were any more fit or leaner.

- In a study from Duke University, depressed people were treated with antidepressant medications, exercise or both. After 16 weeks, up to 70% of all the subjects were no longer depressed. However, the best results came from exercise, while one in three of the patients who took only the medication experienced no relief from depression. Of those who did get some relief from medication, many had adverse side effects from the drugs.

- In another study from Duke University of depressed people who either exercised or took antidepressant medications or placebos, mood lifted in the exercising groups almost as much as in the medication group, with no cost or side effects.

These and other studies do not negate the importance of seeking medical help for clinically diagnosed depression. Always talk to your doctor if you can't rise above the blues. But they do emphasize the importance of including daily activity in treatment, whether or not you need medication, counseling or other medical attention.

You Were Meant to Move

This might come as a surprise, but it's not that physical activity is healthy or good for us. You wouldn't say that oxygen or the basic drive to survive is "good for you."

The lesson here is that our bodies were meant to move. When we don't move, the system breaks down.

Our bodies evolved over millions of years to be vigorously active. It has only been in recent years that we have switched first from being hunter-gatherers to farmers and laborers and now to butt-sitters. When we work against our system's basic need to move, our bodies begin to wither—mentally, emotionally and physically. Compare a couch potato who works against this essential need to move to a gym rat who works with it, and the potato is more than twice as likely to be blue, while it is practically impossible for anyone who is passionately active to have more than an occasional bad day.

Better yet, the move-and-mood link is cyclical. Say you don't feel like exercising, but you lace up your shoes and go for a one-hour walk every day anyway. The likelihood is that within no time your mood will lift, which gives you the incentive to exercise more, which further improves your mood. Before you know it, you've lost weight, are superproud of yourself, have sparked your confidence and lifted your mood, all because you made that initial effort to get some fresh air!

The Self-Confidence Tango

Looking for a shot in the arm of self-confidence? Need a little more self-esteem? Want a *natural high* to be proud of yourself about? Take a dance class. Or jump on the exercise bandwagon of your choice. People who are physically active every day have much better self-images, are more confident and score higher on assessments of self-esteem than are sedentary folks. The more they exercise, the greater their confidence.

Alex, the college student in the Pacific Northwest, has found a source of self-esteem, as well as an energizing habit in exercise:

> "I could not survive without exercise. I take an aerobics class and I also head to the gym at least twice a week, but it's weight lifting that makes me feel the best. My energy, mood and ability to function all benefit from working out. I have lost a lot of weight in the past few years, and along with eating better, exercise makes me feel good about myself and how hard I have worked to get to this leaner, happier, healthier me."

Jog Your Memory

"I feel the mental fog lift when I exercise. I am most invigorated, alive and myself again when I've laced up my jogging shoes and hit the road," says Whitney, a public relations executive in San Francisco. "I have to exercise, otherwise I gain weight. Being physical also puts me in a better mood—after a long run or a good workout session, problems seem to evaporate. It helps me unwind from the stress at the office and it stimulates my creative juices. I think much more clearly on the days when I've gotten off my lazy butt and exercised."

Exercise stimulates blood flow to the brain, supplying it with a hefty dose of oxygen and nutrients. It also minimizes plaque buildup inside blood vessels, so blood flows unhindered. Exercise raises levels of natural substances, called neurotropins, that enhance brain cell growth and help nerve cells process information. Neurotransmitter levels, in particular dopamine, endorphins, serotonin and norepinephrine (which helps in memory storage and retrieval), also increase as much as 29% with exercise.

"When running, I get my best ideas. I call them my 'aha' moments, because solutions to nagging problems, like how to handle a difficult problem with one of my kids or how to talk to my boss about a raise, just pop into my head while I'm jogging," says Julie, a human resources manager in Mill Valley, California.

Convert couch potatoes into exercisers and they show dramatic improvements in thinking ability, reaction times, memory and concentration. They score higher on tests of reaction times, nonverbal reasoning and memory. In fact, they regain the quick-wittedness of youth, no matter what their age. In short, exercise is the ultimate antiaging *natural high* for your brain.

Walk off Stress

People who exercise regularly report less stress, are calmer and handle stress better than sedentary folks. Researchers disagree on whether strenuous or moderate exercise is the best, but they agree that the more exercise you do, the better.

Exercise helps block much of the damaging effects of stress on the brain and body. Elevated stress hormones, like cortisol, are linked to depression, memory loss, tissue damage and weight gain. Exercise "burns up" that damaging cortisol, so you don't stew in your own juices. Over time, the body learns to react less intensely to stress, thus providing a built-in coping mechanism against anxiety.

By de-stressing your life, you also boost brain power. Cortisol interferes with the brain's ability to use glucose, the primary source of fuel for the brain. The resulting energy shortage inhibits the brain's ability to store memories and slows mental function. Cortisol also blocks nerve chemical activity, so your brain can't effectively relay information. Finally, cortisol kills brain cells by disrupting brain cell activity, slowing removal of waste products from brain cells and generating excessive amounts of free radicals. As a result, reaction times, memory, creative thinking and concentration take a nosedive. Daily exercise helps sidestep all that stress-induced damage, leaving you mentally fit as a fiddle.

Exercise can get you through life's toughest moments. Janice, a mother and TV producer in Portland, Oregon, used exercise to get her through a painful divorce. "The doctor wanted to put me on antidepressants, but I wasn't comfortable with that idea, so I kept running. Not only did it calm my nerves and keep me sane during an insane phase of my life, but I ended up being fit enough to run a marathon!"

The same holds true for Bill, a retired social worker in San Diego. "When my wife developed breast cancer, the only thing that got me through those tough times was running. I'd go from a 10 on the stress scale to a 1 after a good run. Exercise then helped me through the grieving process when she died." What began as a way to de-stress became a passion. Twenty years later and in his seventies, Bill has run hundreds of 10Ks and several marathons from the West Coast to the East, including the Boston Marathon.

Pedal Away Fatigue

When you're tired, worn-out from a long day of chasing kids or slaving away on the job, the last thing you might think you need is a good old-fashioned workout. But that is exactly what will put the spring back in your step.

After graduating from college with a degree in accounting, Jill learned that the dreaded tax season and the long Oregon winters were a one-way ticket to fatigue:

"I accepted a position with a large international accounting firm. When the busy season hit in January, for the first time I had trouble balancing my life. The less I did with my personal time, the more tired I felt. My priorities outside of work centered around showering, eating and sleeping. I awoke tired in the morning and shuffled through the day with my eyes half opened. When I returned home from work late at night, I barely made it to my bed before falling asleep. I had never experienced such complete exhaustion. I couldn't imagine doing anything with my free time other than catching every available second of sleep."

Jill's energy level spiraled into a never-ending battle with fatigue until one mid-February night, she hit rock bottom. "I left work around midnight and the next thing

I remember is waking in the morning fully clothed, with my workbag over my shoulder and my shoes still on. I had no memory of driving home or walking up the two flights of stairs to my bedroom." Jill realized she needed to do something to get control of her life again.

Instead of another night collapsing on the bed, she headed down the street to the gym after work:

"I spent 30 minutes on the treadmill, lifted some hand weights and then drove home. The next morning, instead of having to pry my eyes open, I woke before the alarm went off and tackled the beautiful February morning with a quick jog around the neighborhood. I began scheduling 20 to 30 minutes of exercise into my prework schedule, and soon the dread I felt about going to work lifted. Even my friends and coworkers noticed the difference in me."

Jill had been tired and thought she needed more sleep, but it was exercise her body, mind and mood really craved.

Adding movement to your day can boost energy by 20% or more and reduce fatigue up to 65%, even in people who think they are too pooped to pedal. Daily exercisers also feel the most energetic, while the sedentary get drowsier. In one study, people rated their energy levels after 12 days of either eating a candy bar or walking briskly for 10 minutes. Those who walked reported increased energy levels and lowered tension, while those who ate the sugary snack had temporarily raised energy levels, but that high was followed by a crash, with more fatigue and tension.

Along with enhancing body chemistry and reducing stress hormones, exercise lowers blood pressure, fills the lungs and tissues with oxygen and increases levels of adenosine triphosphate (ATP), the high-energy substances generated in our body cells. Stretching also relieves muscle tension that comes from fatigue-producing stress hormones, and it helps move blood throughout the body and oxygenate the brain. In short, if you want more energy, you need to move more every single day.

Move Like an Athlete, Sleep Like a Baby

A major difference between good and bad sleepers may not be what they do at bedtime, but what they did all day. You guessed it—good sleepers are more likely to be physically active. The physical activity helps them cope with daily stress, produces a surge in sleep hormones and tires the body so it is ready to sleep at night.

Exercise also counteracts daytime grogginess that results from not sleeping well by raising calcium levels in the brain, which turns on brain dopamine production and improves mood and energy level. In a study from the University of Washington, people who exercised vigorously for 45 minutes at least three times a week got 33% more deep sleep than did people who were relatively inactive. In another study from Stanford University, healthy adults with mild sleep problems who exercised for at least 40 minutes a day, twice a week, fell asleep faster and slept about 45 minutes longer than people who didn't exercise.

Just Do It

Anyone who sincerely wants to lose weight and keep it off has to move. No ifs, ands or buts. I don't care how old you are, how out of shape, how busy or how stressed. I don't care if your knees hurt, your back has been giving you trouble or you have blisters on your feet. I don't care if there is nowhere to exercise, no one to do it with or you were born without willpower. I don't even care if you eat perfectly, already are at an ideal weight, think you are insanely healthy or assume your low-calorie diet is all it takes to lose weight. Everyone must move. I'm not telling you anything you don't already know. You and everyone within a million-mile radius knows moving is absolutely critical to mood, health and a reasonable waistline.

While any type of daily activity is better than nothing, your best weekly workout plan is one that includes two basic rules:

Basic Rule #1: Exercise almost every day, including two of the following three options:

- *Aerobic activity:* walking, swimming, dancing, kickboxing, jogging, etc
- *Strength training:* lifting weights, doing Pilates or calisthenics, such as sit-ups
- *Warm-up and cool-down:* flexibility movements, yoga, etc

That three-part mix maximizes the mood- and energy-lifting effects of physical activity, reduces the risk for injury and increases both the chances that you won't get bored and that you will live long, happy and well.

Basic Rule #2: Move more throughout the day. Besides your planned exercise, strap on a pedometer and aim for that magic 10,000 steps a day. Even if you miss the mark and total only 4,000 steps a day, you still will lose 5 pounds or more in a year.

Tallying 10,000 steps isn't that hard. Walk up and down the hallway while you brush your teeth or talk on the phone. Walk the aisles at work while you ponder the solution to a problem. Make a pact with yourself to only watch TV when walking the treadmill.

Must I Sweat?

The level of intensity and even the type of exercise doesn't seem to matter. Intense and moderate activities, as well as aerobic activities, such as walking, running or swimming; or anaerobic sports, such as bodybuilding, all alleviate depression and improve mood.

Noncompetitive sports, like aerobic dance, swimming laps or riding an exercise bicycle, and exercises that are repetitive and predictable, such as running the same wooded trail up and back, appear to offer the best mood boost. The best exercise routine, however, is the one you will stick with and enjoy the most.

Even a little bit of mild exercise is enough to lift mood. One study from the University of Alabama found that just a 30-minute walk every day had an amazing effect on lifting mood. Another study from Stanford University found that low-intensity exercise was just as good as high-intensity for lowering disease risk. Better yet, those who worked out at home were just as fit as those who went to the gym, and they were more likely to stick with it! Of course, exercise is only effective at boosting mood if you do it every day. Depression can return within 48 hours of not exercising.

When it comes to maximizing brain power, the type of exercise you choose might make a difference. Stretching and toning exercises are great for your muscles and your bones, and they help with flexibility and balance. They even lower stress. But they aren't the best for thinking, memory and multitasking. Aerobic activities, such as walking, swimming, running or cross-country skiing, help boost thinking ability, probably because they pump extra oxygen into brain tissue and also enhance the brain chemistry designed to help you think fast and smart. A combination of aerobics and weight lifting will give you the best gains in mental power.

Get with It

If you are not used to daily exercise, then you'll need to set some ground rules before jumping into an exercise routine.

First, you must *make it a priority.* Write it in your daily calendar as if it were a dentist appointment, then let nothing get in the way of that schedule. Plan ahead. Bring exercise clothes to work or when traveling. At home, put on your exercise clothes when you get up in the morning or when you arrive home after work; keep them on until you've exercised. Remember: failing to plan is planning to fail.

Second, put your weight-loss goals on hold in the beginning. For the first six months, focus on fitting exercise into your busy schedule, and pay attention to the mood and energy changes. Studies show that people who exercise to feel energized and happy are the ones most likely to stick with their programs. Their workouts give them an instant payoff by improving their day, and the long-term benefits motivate them to stick with it. The weight loss will happen, possibly even effortlessly, but don't make it a priority at first.

Third, define yourself as someone who is active. Look for excuses to exercise rather than reasons why you can't. Spend time with people who exercise, or join a gym. The shift in attitude happens gradually, but it will slowly transform how you view yourself and your relationship with exercise, which in turn will help motivate you to stick with it.

Do This

Of course, rousing an out-of-shape body off the couch and into the gym won't feel as good as, say, polishing off a few Krispy Kremes—at least, not at first. You must move enough to see benefits (that means you must sweat), but not so much that soreness or fatigue get in the way of motivation.

To get the mood and energy-lifting results without feeling awful, gradually increase the duration, intensity or frequency of your exercise session. Those who stick with an exercise program for at least six months—even those who admit they had been exercise phobic—say that if they had only known how good they would feel, they would have started exercising earlier!

A rule of thumb is to increase time or intensity by 10% each week. If you're currently walking 1 mile a day, increase the distance to 1.1 miles the next week and do it in the same amount of time. Also, add other activities to the program as you advance. Your ultimate goal is to accumulate at least 30, and preferably 60, minutes or more every day of moderate-intensity activity.

Mix it up with some walking or other aerobic activity, some muscle-building activity like Pilates, and some stretching/balancing like yoga. Then commit to making it fun.

Don't Do This

Along with all the "do's" are a few "don'ts" when it comes to exercise.

- **Don't sabotage your efforts.** The biggest mistake people make when starting an exercise program is they try to do too much too soon. They work out with vigor at the gym that they are so sore the next day they can't move. By week's end, the exercise shoes are at the back of the closet.
- **Don't overdo it.** Develop a program that is well within your ability. That way, early success will encourage long-term commitment. If you know you can walk 15 minutes at a brisk pace, walk only 10 minutes each day the first week. You won't feel sore and will be encouraged to stick with your program.
- **Don't make it hurt.** Exercise doesn't have to hurt to be good for you. Brisk walking (at

a pace that allows you to cover 2 miles in less than half an hour) is the number one activity that diet successes in the National Weight Control Registry have adopted, and it's the most frequently chosen exercise to boost mood and energy level.

Move It, Baby, Move It

You have listened to me rant and rave through this entire book about the importance of good food and the right nutrients to improve your mood and slim your waistline. All of that is absolutely true. What, when and how much you eat will have a profound effect on how much you enjoy life as well as how quickly you lose weight.

But let's get real. Blueberries are not the cure-all for depression, stress, fatigue, memory loss or sleep problems. Yes, berries or sweet potatoes or oranges will help protect your brain from stress and a blue mood, but no food holds a candle to the benefits you will get from exercising daily.

Read my lips: you can't get to happy and fit by food alone. But combine those blueberries, carrots, other real foods and the rest of the advice in this book with a commitment to exercise almost every day and for the rest of your life, and I promise you will feel, think, look and be the best you have ever been in your life. Just take the advice of Susan, a waitress in Dallas:

"I used to think I'd be happy if I just won the lottery or found 'Mr. Wonderful,' or even if 'Mr. Paycheck' came along. But I've read those stories in magazines about how the lives of lottery winners are messed up by money, and I've had my fair share of Mr. Rights and Mr. Wrongs and none of them made me happy forever. I finally realized about five years ago, that if I wanted to be really happy, it was up to me to make my dreams come true. Since then, I've cleaned up my diet act. I don't like to walk for exercise, since I walk so much for my job already. So, I joined an aerobics class and also fell in love with mountain biking. Once I took charge of my life, owned my decisions and started treating myself with a little respect by taking care of my health, it was crystal clear that the only one who can make me happy is me. And now I am!"

SECRETS REVEALED:
PUTTING IT ALL TOGETHER

All the secrets of happy, fit people are on the table. Now you know everything there is to know, based on tried-and-true, time-tested, proven habits about what, when and how happy, fit people eat to maximize their chances for being blissfully thin—or at least much happier, more energetic, less stressed and a whole lot leaner. You now know what successful dieters and joyful people do every day to guarantee they lose weight, keep it off and stay upbeat and energized through the process.

Adopt some of the habits, guidelines, tips and secrets from this book and you will feel better than you've ever felt in your life. I am always amazed at how grateful the body and mind are for a little tender loving care.

Recently, after giving a presentation on food and mood at a women's conference in Kentucky, a woman came up to me eager to tell her story:

"I changed doctors last year and my new doctor told me that if I refused to eat well, that she refused to see me. Wow. What an eye-opener.

It dawned on me that if I wasn't going to meet my doctor halfway by taking care of myself, why should I take it for granted that she would even want me as a patient? It was the wake-up call I needed. I changed my eating habits, adopting many of the tips you suggested in your presentation this morning, and within weeks, I started feeling so much better. My mood improved, my energy level got a shot in the arm and I'm even sleeping better. I've also lost 37 pounds, and still counting. What you eat really does make a huge difference in how you feel!"

Of course, there are a few ground rules to getting back in touch with your blissfully thin inner self. You must

- **Believe you deserve it.** You must believe you are worthy of being cared for, just as you care for others. You need your own time and space to care for yourself. You deserve that time and that care to be the happiest, healthiest and leanest person you were meant to be. When you are happy, that happiness will spread to others. This isn't a selfish wish; it's one goal that will keep on giving.

- **Decide you want it.** You need to really want happiness and health. You must want this for yourself, not because anyone says you need it or wants you to have it. You must want it, and you must want it bad, for your health, your self-respect and your future. You are absolutely right, it isn't fair that some people must move more or eat less than others, but that's the reality. It's time to accept that managing your weight, your mood and your health is a lifelong process within your power.

You also must accept there are no magic pills, no diet gurus, no gizmos or gadgets that can do it for you.

- **Get started.** Make a plan, decide on your strategies, then set to work. If a strategy doesn't pan out, tweak your plan and keep going. Take it one meal, one day, one week and one month at a time. As Winston Churchill said, "Never, never, never give up!"

- **Keep at it.** You will slip. Everyone does. To think you won't slip is like expecting to win a gold medal at the Olympics without training. The trick is to not let a slip escalate to a relapse. People who successfully maintain weight loss are vigilant in their efforts. They essentially nip weight regain in the bud, day by day and meal by meal. Although the method varies, maintainers know that setbacks are inevitable and they have attack plans in place to quickly handle slips. They weigh themselves regularly (once a week or more), keep records of their food intake and return to their mood-improving or weight-loss efforts at the first sign of a slip. The good news is that maintainers consistently report that it gets easier over time. It's a practice makes perfect scenario. The longer you keep at it, the more natural it gets.

What Would You Do Differently?

Imagine yourself blissfully happy, at peace with yourself and your loved ones and proud of your body and life. What would you do differently if you really and truly believed each of the following statements?

I believe:	If this was really true, I would:
I deserve to be blissfully happy.	_____
I can do anything I set my mind to do.	_____
My goals and dreams are important.	_____
I deserve to eat well and be fit.	_____
I am valuable and important.	_____
I can succeed at weight loss.	_____
I can be happy and healthy.	_____

Where Do I Start?

Eating right doesn't begin in the kitchen or even at the supermarket. It starts with a plan. That plan must fit your routine and include your food preferences, as well as garner support from family, coworkers, friends or anyone else who influences your eating and exercise habits.

Sit down with yourself, pen in hand, and get honest. Brutally honest. What diet habits need the most change?

- If you skip breakfast but then overeat later in the day, maybe it is a plan that lays out exactly what and how much you will eat in the morning, as explained in Chapter 2.
- If you are a carb junkie, then your plan might start by clearing your cupboards of the processed junk, as mentioned in Chapter 3.
- If your sweet tooth gets the better of you, then defining a plan how you will cut back on added sugar, while maximizing the sweetness of antioxidant-rich fruits might be the first place to start. Chapter 4 will give you more than enough ideas on how to do that.
- Do you already eat fairly well and just need to kick your nutrition up a notch by adding more super mood foods to the daily fare? Then the ideas in Chapter 5 will be the basis of your plan.

- A plan to include more of the omega-3 fat DHA could be the target if you seldom eat salmon or are concerned about your memory today and down the road. Chapter 6 gives you lots of foods fortified with this fat, as well as some ideas how to boost intake with the best seafood.

- Looking for a total overhaul on your supplement plan? Chapter 7 gives you lots of ideas about which nutrients to focus on and how to choose the best multivitamin.

- If happy hour is undermining your mood and waistline, then Chapter 8 is the place to look for ideas on how to quench your thirst without sacrificing your figure.

- If your weakness is giving in to cravings, then start with Chapter 9 on how to rein in your vices.

- If a good night's sleep eludes you, then Chapter 10 might be where you start in your plan to feel and look your best.

- Finally, if your diet already is perfect, but you need a good kick in the you-know-what when it comes to mood-boosting, fat-burning exercise, then the bonus chapter on how to move for your mood is just the ticket.

The Plan

Ask any happy, fit person how they got started and you are likely to hear something about keeping a food diary. Jotting down what, how much and when you eat, even if only for a few days, provides priceless feedback on what eating habits are blocking your road to bliss. People who reach their goals and, more important, maintain the change, say that keeping a food diary was their single most important strategy.

Jot down what, how much and when you eat for three to seven days. Then look back over your records, checking for patterns or surprises. Perhaps your records show that the more chocolate you eat, the more you want (a sign of sugar addiction), or that your typical vegetable intake is a lot less than you thought. These eye-openers are the beginning of your plan.

The next step is to create a plan to solve the problem. Your plan might be to remove chocolate temptations from your house or to satisfy a chocolate craving three times a week, but not every day. A plan to include more colorful produce might start with a vow to include at least two at every meal.

Putting know-how into action requires having the tools to get there.

- For breakfast ideas, turn to Chapter 2.
- Lunch ideas to keep you energized throughout the afternoon can be found in Chapter 1.
- Snooze-promoting dinners are found in Chapter 10.
- Snack ideas are in Chapter 3.

- Looking for ways to quench your thirst for few calories? Then turn to Chapter 8.
- For desserts that give your energy and mood a lift, check out Chapter 9.
- At a loss as to how to shop for both your mood and your figure? Then use the shopping list on page 15 in Chapter 1 and the partial list of processed foods that meet the real-foods guidelines in the Appendix on page 425.
- Want a specific plan on how to incorporate real food and super mood foods into your diet? Then try the two weeks' worth of menus starting on page 387.
- If you're tired of the same old same old, then get adventuresome with the super foods in the Recipes section. It's all here and ready for the taking.

Whatever your plan, it only will work if you stick with it. It needs to be as realistic and simple as possible. After keeping a food diary for a few days and identifying one or two habits that are out of whack with those of people who are happy and lean, then take those "bad" habits and brainstorm solutions. Write down every solution that comes to mind, no matter how silly or far-fetched. If you realize you overeat cookies, crackers and other highly processed junk food when watching TV, your brainstorming list could include,

- Throw all those temptations away.
- Make a vow never to enter the kitchen after 8:00 p.m.
- Lock those foods in a cabinet and only let your spouse know the combination.
- Portion the tempting foods into 1-ounce baggies.
- Use TV time to exercise instead of eat.
- Find a replacement food, such as a cup of tea and two ginger snaps.

Arrange the list according to priorities, starting with the ones that contribute the most to the problem, will have the greatest impact and are realistic for you. Maybe you know yourself well enough to realize you can't steer clear of the kitchen all night, and you know you can't trust your spouse to keep the combination a secret. That whittles the list down to tossing the temptations, portioning a few into baggies, getting an exercise bike or trying a replacement. Pick one or two and make a plan.

Your plan must be realistic. If you know anyone who has gone on a really silly fad diet, like the cabbage soup diet or some ridiculous food-combining diet, you know that they always, always, always end in failure. That's because they aren't realistic. You can't eat cabbage soup for the rest of your life, just as you can't obsess over exactly what will and what won't work together on a plate.

When designing the steps in your plan, ask yourself, "Can I live with this forever? Is this a change I can fit in to my and my family's daily routine?" A plan is only as good as its fit with your life. The best plan in the world is worthless if it doesn't work for your lifestyle. Keep an open mind and experiment with different strategies and tactics. Just because one doesn't work doesn't mean you've lost the game. It only means you haven't yet found the strategy or plan that works best for you.

Your plan also must be very specific. No loopholes, no excuses, no wiggle room allowed! Let's say your problem is you always end up ordering a 700-calorie blueberry muffin whenever you stop at a coffee shop for your morning java. Your plan could be to

1. have a quick-fix breakfast at home that follows the 1-2-3 Rule, then
2. take a different route to work so you aren't tempted to pull in for a second breakfast.

That plan is easy to track. You know exactly what you must do. You also know exactly when you do and don't stay on track.

You aren't a failure if your plan doesn't work at first. This is a work in progress. Some plans work, others don't. You are experimenting, looking for the plan that fits in to your lifestyle.

Take, for example, the plan to eat breakfast and drive a different route. You might find that you don't always find time for breakfast at home, so you arrive at work hungry and more tempted by the office dough-nuts. Time to tweak your plan. Try instead to stock your desk and the employee fridge with individual boxes of cereal, cartons of milk and fresh fruit. Then have a desk-fast when you get to work while check-ing your email. Measure your progress continually with stars on a calendar, marks on a list, points on a scorecard or whatever works for you.

Your diet does not exist in a vacuum. It's part of your entire life. You need to create a plan that embraces the bigger picture. Information gathered from your food diary will help identify the things that contribute to your nutrition, exercise or mood and weight problem. Maybe you realize that when you spend time with the neighbor next door, you are much more likely to eat junk food and sit around discussing movie star gossip or baseball scores. That means your bigger picture needs to include more friends who support your new lifestyle and who like to walk while they chat. Keep experimenting with solutions until you find one or more that solve the problem.

The New You

Your ultimate goal is to be the happiest, healthiest and leanest you can be. There are no quick-fix solutions to that goal. There is no one food or one habit that is the solution to all your ills. Instead, it is a continuous process of improving yourself. A process that takes a lifetime. To stop improving yourself is to die.

I hope that process includes joy. Realize, too, that bringing happiness into your life may require some changes. The more changes you make toward being the happiest and leanest you, the more dramatic the results. Any change, no matter how small, is one step closer to your true blissful self. Go for it! Don't settle for less than your best! I promise you the payoffs are well worth it.

14-DAY
KICK-START DIET FOR A GOOD MOOD

Here is two weeks' worth of happy meals that help you say "bye-bye" to the blues and an extra pound or two by putting into practice the diet rules for feeling great. Days 8 and 14 allow you to try out the new recipes in the Recipes section. The 200-calorie snacks are designed for either a midafternoon or late-night snack to boost serotonin levels and both curb cravings and help you sleep. They are optional and can be omitted if you are not hungry between meals or want to lose an extra 2 ½ pounds each month. While these menus are a perfect plan for eating right, boosting your mood and slimming your waistline, it is difficult to meet all of your vitamin and mineral needs on less than 1,800 calories a day, so make sure to take a well-formulated multivitamin and mineral supplement to fill in any nutrient gaps.

DAY 1

Breakfast

Two frozen whole-wheat waffles, toasted and topped with 3 tablespoons fat-free sour cream and ⅔ cup fresh or thawed blueberries

6 ounces 100% grapefruit or orange juice

Herb tea (optional)

Lunch

Half a turkey sandwich made from one slice whole-wheat bread, 2 ounces turkey breast and 1 tablespoon cranberry sauce

Spinach salad made with 2 cups fresh chopped spinach, sliced mushrooms, 2 tablespoons fresh red raspberries and 2 tablespoons fat-free raspberry vinaigrette dressing

1 tangerine, peeled and sectioned

Sparkling water with lime

Dinner

Pasta with Tomatoes and Clams: 1 cup cooked whole-wheat pasta topped with a sauce: ½ cup chopped onion, 8 ounces stewed tomatoes,

2 teaspoons chopped fresh parsley, two minced garlic cloves, ½ teaspoon marjoram, salt and pepper simmered in a nonstick skillet until onion is tender. Add ¼ pound fresh shelled steamer clams and cook for 10 minutes over medium-high heat. Pour over pasta.

1 cup steamed broccoli

Tomatoes with Mozzarella and Basil: Cut a medium tomato into three slices and top each slice with a thin slice of fresh mozzarella cheese and a fresh basil leaf. Drizzle 2 teaspoons low-fat balsamic vinaigrette dressing over the slices.

One mango, peeled and sliced and topped with 6 ounces nonfat lemon yogurt and chopped mint leaves

This meal is filling, but not overly heavy, so it won't interfere with a good night's sleep. The carbs will help boost serotonin, so you will be more apt to sleep well and awaken refreshed and energized tomorrow.

200-Calorie, All-Carb Snack

⅔ cup Cheerios, 4 tablespoons dried cranberries and 1 tablespoon candied ginger. Serve with water.

Nutritional information without snack: 1,590 calories, 19% fat (33.6 g total, 11 g saturated); 23% protein (91 g), 58% carbs (231 g), 28 g fiber, 1,071 mg calcium, 479 mcg folate, 1,474 mg sodium

Nutritional information with snack: 1,800 calories, 17% fat (34 g total, 11 g saturated), 21% protein (94.5 g), 62% carbs (279 g), 32 g fiber; 1,117 mg calcium; 484 mcg folate; 1,643 mg sodium

DAY 2

Breakfast

Two eggs, scrambled with ¼ cup diced red peppers and 2 tablespoons diced onion

[Eggs: choose ones that contain DHA from a plant source, contaminant-free omega-3, such as Gold Circle Farm eggs, to boost brain and mood.]

One slice 100% whole-wheat toast topped with 1 teaspoon butter

One medium tomato, sliced

1 cup low-fat milk with DHA

Green tea (optional)

To help restock glucose stores, brain levels of a nerve chemical called neuropeptide Y (NPY) are high in the morning, which trigger preferences for the best source of glucose—grains. Work with NPY by taking time to eat a carb-rich breakfast and you will be less prone to emotional eating later in the day.

Lunch

One Black Bean Burrito: Fill a whole-wheat tortilla with ⅓ cup drained black beans, 1 ounce low-fat cheese (such as Cabot Vermont 50% Reduced-Fat cheddar cheese with DHA), three slices avocado, 2 tablespoons chopped fresh cilantro and 2 tablespoons salsa.

One sliced red bell pepper

A great alternative to typical crunchy snacks! Most commercial crispy snacks are greasy, salty and nutrient-poor. The salt dehydrates the body, leading to fatigue. Instead, if you are feeling stressed and need something to sink your teeth into, munch on crunchy fruits and vegetables, such as red pepper slices.

Ten baby carrots

1 tablespoon low-fat ranch dressing

2 small oatmeal cookies

1 cup low-fat milk with DHA

The combination of milk and dessert might raise levels of endorphins, morphinelike compounds in the brain that produce a euphoric feeling.

Dinner

One 4-ounce grilled chicken breast, marinated in wine, garlic and herbs

⅔ cup green peas and carrots, steamed

Half an acorn squash, baked and drizzled with 1 teaspoon honey and ½ teaspoon rum extract

Tossed salad made from 2 cups deep-green lettuce, half a winter pear cut into slivers and 2 tablespoons fat-free vinaigrette

Fruit and Chocolate Fondue: Dunk 1 cup fresh strawberries and one peeled and sliced kiwi in ¼ cup fat-free chocolate syrup.

Chocolate is the number one most-craved food. It also contains brain chemicals, such as phenylethylamine and anandamide that mimic the feeling of being in love. Keep yourself happy without sacrificing your waistline with this yummy dessert.

200-Calorie, All-Carb Snack

Half a whole-wheat bagel, toasted and topped with 1 tablespoon fat-free sour cream and 1 teaspoon all-fruit jam. Serve with water.

Nutritional information without snack: 1,605 calories, 24% fat (43 g total, 12 g saturated), 23% protein (92 g), 53% carbs (213 g), 35 g fiber, 1,157 mg calcium, 544 mcg folate, 1,902 mg sodium

Nutritional information with snack: 1,795 calories, 24% fat (48 g total,
16 g saturated), 22% protein (99 g), 54% carbs (242 g), 38 g fiber,
1,203 mg calcium, 577 mcg folate, 2,133 mg sodium

DAY 3

Breakfast

1 cup cooked old-fashioned oatmeal, cooked in 1 cup
low-fat milk and topped with 2 tablespoons toasted
wheat germ and 1 tablespoon brown sugar

One banana, sliced and sprinkled with cinnamon

6 ounces calcium-fortified orange juice

Green tea

Lunch

Pita sandwich made with one whole-wheat pita,
1 ounce jalapeño Jack cheese, one medium
diced tomato, ½ cup drained kidney beans and
3 tablespoons chopped fresh cilantro.

*Whole grains enter the bloodstream slowly, thus
preventing the rapid rise and fall of blood sugar
levels that can leave you feeling jittery, irritable and
craving carbs.*

One medium orange, peeled and sectioned

Iced herb tea

Dinner

4 ounces grilled salmon, seasoned with lemon juice and fresh dill

15 asparagus spears, lightly steamed and sprinkled with red pepper flakes

1 cup yellow squash rounds, lightly steamed

½ cup whole-grain couscous, prepared according to package

1 cup steamed low-fat milk with DHA, flavored with ½ teaspoon almond extract

1 cup grapes

Salmon is one of the best natural sources of the omega-3 fats, which help keep your mood on an even keel. The asparagus is an excellent source of the brain-boosting B vitamin folate.

200-Calorie, All-Carb Snack

⅔ cup berry sorbet topped with 1 cup raspberries. Serve with water.

Satisfy dwindling serotonin levels and your sweet tooth midday or after dinner with this all-carb snack.

Nutritional information without snack: 1,612 calories, 21% fat (37 g total, 15 g saturated), 22% protein (89 g), 57% carbs (230 g), 36 g fiber, 1,319 mg calcium, 727 mcg folate, 785 mg sodium

Nutritional information with snack: 1,796 calories, 19% fat (38 g total, 15 g saturated), 20% protein (90 g), 61% carbs (274 g), 41 g fiber, 1,352 mg calcium, 765 mcg folate, 804 mg sodium

DAY 4

Breakfast

One 3-ounce whole-wheat bran muffin topped with 1 tablespoon peanut butter

½ cup fresh or canned pineapple chunks

1 cup soy milk with DHA, steamed and flavored with cinnamon and Nutrasweet

Lunch

Zesty Grilled Cheese Sandwich: Grill the following sandwich using vegetable spray: two slices 100% whole-wheat bread; 1 ounce low-fat cheddar cheese; one large canned green chili, drained; one medium tomato, sliced.

1 ½ cups reduced-sodium vegetable soup (per directions on can)

Carrot salad made with ⅔ cup grated carrots, 1 tablespoon raisins, 2 tablespoons fat-free mayonnaise, 1 teaspoon lemon juice, and salt and pepper to taste

6 ounces low-fat milk with DHA

A light lunch, such as this one, keeps you energized during the afternoon and helps avoid that sluggish feeling, both mental and physical, that results from eating a heavy, fatty or calorie-packed lunch.

Dinner

Mango Chutney Chicken: Top a 4-ounce grilled chicken breast with a mixture of 3 tablespoons Major Grey's Chutney and ¼ cup diced mango

½ cup steamed fresh green beans

1 cup tossed salad with 1 tablespoon low-calorie dressing

One small slice angel food cake topped with ½ cup fresh strawberries

A little something sweet can boost levels of endorphins, the same feel-good chemicals that produce a runner's high.

200-Calorie, All-Carb Snack

People who divide their food intake into little meals and snacks evenly spaced throughout the day work with their appetite centers, which helps avoid fatigue, mood swings and uncontrollable cravings. On the other hand, snacking on cookies or pop will

undermine your mood and energy. Both when and what you eat is important.

1 cup air-popped popcorn flavored with a dash of hot pepper sauce

1 papaya, seeded and drizzled with 1 teaspoon fresh lime juice

Nutritional information without snack: 1,595 calories, 27% fat (48 g total, 16 g saturated), 20% protein (80 g), 53% carbs (211 g), 25 g fiber, 1,098 mg calcium, 307 mcg folate, 4,014 mg sodium

Nutritional information with snack: 1,806 calories, 24% fat (48 g total, 16 g saturated), 18% protein (81 g), 58% carbs (262 g), 37 g fiber, 1,174 mg calcium, 428 mcg folate, 4,024 mg sodium

DAY 5

Breakfast

Make-Ahead Breakfast: The night before, mix ⅔ cup low-fat granola and ⅔ cup soy milk in a bowl. Place in refrigerator. In the morning, add half a diced green apple (such as Granny Smith) and mix. Top with half a banana, sliced.

Low-fat Latte: Dark-roasted coffee and ⅔ cup warmed low-fat milk with DHA

Lunch

Tuna Salad Sandwich: 3 ounces drained tuna packed in water, ¼ cup chopped celery, 1 tablespoon diced red onion, 1 teaspoon mustard, 2 tablespoons low-fat mayonnaise, dried dill and pepper to taste and lettuce on two slices 100% whole-wheat bread.

Tomato-Corn Salad: Mix two chopped tomatoes, ⅓ cup corn kernels, 2 tablespoons diced red onion and 2 teaspoons chopped cilantro with rice wine vinegar and salt to taste.

1 cup broccoli florets dunked in 2 tablespoons low-fat ranch dressing

Diets low in folate are linked with depression and memory loss, while optimal intake of this B vitamin improves mood, attention and mental function. This crunchy broccoli and dip is a folate-packed munchable.

Sparkling water with a lemon slice

Dinner

3 ounces grilled flank steak

One 4-ounce baked sweet potato topped with chives and 2 tablespoons fat-free sour cream

Grilled Vegetables: Coat the following in

2 teaspoons olive oil, garlic powder, salt and pepper
and grill or broil for 5 to 10 minutes, turning
occasionally: ⅓ cup peeled and cubed eggplant,
⅓ cup green bell peppers sliced into ½-inch strips,
½ cup zucchini cut into ½-inch rounds.

1 cup low-fat milk with DHA flavored with
vanilla extract

200-Calorie, All-Carb Snack

Two 100% whole-wheat Fig Newtons

6-ounce glass apricot nectar

Nutritional information without snack: 1,593 calories, 27% fat
(48 g total, 13 g saturated), 22% protein (88 g), 51% carbs (203 g),
29 g fiber, 924 mg calcium, 494 mcg folate, 1,704 mg sodium

Nutritional information with snack: 1,785 calories, 25% fat
(50 g total, 14 g saturated), 20% protein (89 g), 55% carbs (245 g),
31 g fiber, 954 mg calcium, 499 mcg folate, 1,807 mg sodium

DAY 6

Breakfast

Breakfast-in-a-Glass Smoothie: Blend together
1 cup low-fat milk with DHA, ¼ cup toasted
wheat germ, ¾ cup whole-grain flake cereal,
one banana, 2 tablespoons maple syrup and
½ teaspoon maple extract.

Lunch

Lox, Cream Cheese and Bagel: One toasted 100% whole-wheat bagel topped with 3 ounces smoked salmon/lox, 2 tablespoons nonfat cream cheese, one slice red onion, one thick slice tomato and 2 tablespoons alfalfa sprouts.

Ten baby carrots

1 cup tomato juice

Dinner

Juicy, Thick Cheeseburger: 3 ounces grilled or broiled ground turkey breast, 1 ounce reduced-fat cheddar cheese with DHA, one medium sliced tomato, two lettuce leaves, one slice red onion, catsup and mustard to taste and one 100% whole-grain hamburger bun.

Sweet Potato Fries: One medium sweet potato, cut into wedges, sprinkled with salt (if desired), placed on a vegetable-sprayed cookie sheet, and baked at 425 degrees until slightly crispy (about 20 minutes).

The number one vegetable on Americans' plates, French fries, are the least nutritious of any selection in the produce department. Sweet potatoes, on the other hand, are a super mood food, loaded with potassium, beta-carotene, vitamin C, magnesium, fiber and more.

Spinach Salad: 2 ½ cups chopped or baby spinach leaves, 1 tablespoon diced red onion, ¼ cup raspberries and 2 tablespoons fat-free raspberry vinaigrette.

200-Calorie, All-Carb Snack

Open-Face Creamy Peach Sandwich: Blend 2 tablespoons fat-free cream cheese, 1 teaspoon honey and one peach, peeled and chopped. Spread on a slice of 7-grain bread and sprinkle with ½ teaspoon chopped walnuts. Serve with water.

Nutritional information without snack: 1,597 calories, 22% fat (39 g total, 16 g saturated), 22% protein (88 g), 56% carbs (224 g), 33 g fiber, 970 mg calcium, 725 mcg folate, 4,035 mg sodium

Nutritional information with snack: 1,799 calories, 21% fat (42 g total, 16 saturated), 22% protein (99 g), 57% carbs (256 g), 37 g fiber, 1,001 mg calcium, 746 mcg folate, 4,559 mg sodium

DAY 7

Breakfast

Veggie Omelet: Spray a medium skillet with vegetable spray and sauté half a carrot, peeled and thinly sliced; ¼ cup broccoli pieces; and 2 tablespoons sliced yellow onion over medium heat until heated through but still firm. Whip together two medium whole eggs and salt and pepper to taste. Pour over vegetable mixture, top with 1 ounce grated cheddar cheese, cover, reduce heat to medium low, and cook until firm (about 15 minutes).

One piece 100% whole-grain toast with 1 teaspoon butter

Half a grapefruit, broiled (cut grapefruit in half, top with a pinch each of sugar, cinnamon and nutmeg and broil until bubbly)

Café Latte: Coffee with 1 cup warmed low-fat milk with DHA.

A cup of coffee in the morning can help kick-start your energy and attention, just don't go overboard and drink it all day long!

Lunch

Spinach-Chicken Wrap: Fill one whole-wheat tortilla (preferably one fortified with DHA) with 3 ounces grilled or roasted chicken breast, ¼ cup baby spinach leaves, ¼ cup bottled roasted red peppers and 2 tablespoons fat-free cream cheese. Heat in microwave. Top with 2 teaspoons salsa.

1 cup sliced fresh peaches topped with nutmeg

1 cup low-fat milk with DHA

Dinner

3 ounces grilled halibut topped with lemon juice and chopped fresh basil leaves

Green Mashed Potatoes: One 6-ounce baking potato, peeled, boiled and mashed with ⅔ cup steamed chopped chard, 2 teaspoons butter, salt and pepper to taste, and enough fat-free half & half to form a creamy consistency (approximately ⅓ cup).

Sneak greens into your diet to boost folate. Add to soups, stews, lasagna and these mashed potatoes.

Coleslaw: 1 cup preshredded cabbage mixed with ¼ cup drained canned pineapple chunks and 1 tablespoon low-calorie coleslaw dressing

200-Calorie, All-Carb Snack

1 ⅔ cups frozen blueberries and two graham crackers

Nutritional information without snack: 1,604 calories, 30% fat (53 g total, 26 g saturated), 27% protein (108 g), 43% carbs (172 g), 19 g fiber, 1,284 mg calcium, 270 mcg folate, 1,659 mg sodium

Nutritional information with snack: 1,798 calories, 28% fat (56 g total, 26 g saturated), 24% protein (108 g), 48% carbs (216 g), 25 g fiber, 1,302 mg calcium, 288 mcg folate, 1,758 mg sodium

DAY 8

Breakfast

One serving Plum Nuts Oatmeal*

1 cup cantaloupe cubes

Green tea

The combination of deep-orange fruit and nuts is a perfect way to get two super, mood-boosting foods into your daily diet.

Midmorning Snack

One serving Minty Rice, Orange and Pomegranate Bowl*

Sparkling water with lemon

Lunch

One serving Spiced-up Tofu, Orange and Avocado Salad*

1 cup tomato juice

Two slices sourdough French bread

Dinner

Two or three Spicy Salmon Tacos*

1 cup spicy carrots (carrots sliced thin and mixed with jalapeño peppers)

One Poached Pear in Chocolate Lavender Sauce*

Herb tea or decaf coffee

Optional Snack

1 serving Pineapple Coconut Smoothie*

Nutritional information without snacks: 1,953 calories, 19% fat (41 g total, 9 g saturated), 66% carbs (322 g), 15% protein (73 g), 38 g fiber, 962 mg calcium, 492 mcg folate, 1,615 mg sodium

Nutritional information with snacks: 2,193 calories, 19% fat (46 g total, 10 g saturated), 66% carbs (362 g), 15% protein (82 g), 40 g fiber, 1,363 mg calcium, 533 mcg folate, 1,760 mg sodium

DAY 9

Breakfast

Burritoville: Whole-grain tortilla, warmed and filled with: one whole egg and one egg white (or ½ cup egg substitute), scrambled; 1 ounce reduced-fat cheddar cheese; 3 tablespoons salsa; 3 tablespoons chopped tomato; and 3 tablespoons chopped fresh cilantro.

1 cup cubed melon (honeydew, cantaloupe, musk)

Green tea (optional)

Lunch

Spicy Tomato Soup: 1 ½ cups canned healthy tomato soup made with 1% low-fat milk with DHA and topped with ⅓ cup wasabi peas (or edamame and a dash of cayenne pepper).

Grilled Cheese Sandwich: Two slices 100% whole-wheat bread grilled with 1 ½ ounces reduced-fat cheddar cheese with DHA; ¼ cup bottled roasted red peppers, drained; and 1 teaspoon Dijon mustard.

1 cup sparkling water mixed with ¼ cup calcium- and vitamin D-fortified orange juice and crushed ice

Dinner

Lamb Kabobs: Mix 3 tablespoons sherry, 1 teaspoon olive oil and two minced garlic cloves and drizzle over 2 ounces lamb shoulder or leg, cut into cubes; 1 cup zucchini chunks, twelve large mushrooms, ⅓ cup large slices of onion and twelve cherry tomatoes. Marinate for up to eight hours, then skewer and barbecue over medium heat until meat is cooked through, turning occasionally.

1 cup cooked whole-grain couscous

Sautéed Spinach: 6 ounces frozen spinach sautéed with 2 teaspoons olive oil and two minced garlic cloves.

200-Calorie, All-Carb Snack

S'More Snacks: Place four marshmallows and two chocolate Kisses on a graham cracker and top with another graham cracker. Heat in microwave until soft.

Nutritional information without snack: 1,607 calories, 26% fat (46 g total, 12.5 g saturated), 23% protein (92 g), 51% carbs (205 g), 31 g fiber, 1,271 mg calcium, 601 mcg folate, 2,115 mg sodium

Nutritional information with snack: 1,805 calories, 25% fat (50.4 g total, 14.5 g saturated), 20% protein (94 g), 55% carbs (248 g), 31.6 g fiber, 1,294 g calcium, 604 mcg folate, 2,221 mg sodium

DAY 10

Breakfast

Peachy, Creamy Smoothie: Blend 2 tablespoons orange juice concentrate, 1 cup frozen peaches, one banana, 6 ounces low-fat vanilla yogurt, 1 tablespoon toasted wheat germ and a dash of almond extract.

Lunch

Deli-licious Ham Sandwich: Two slices 100% whole-wheat bread, 1 tablespoon Dijon mustard, 3 ounces extra-lean ham and four lettuce leaves.

Coleslaw: 2 ½ cups preshredded cabbage; ⅓ cup canned pineapple chunks, drained; 2 tablespoons low-fat coleslaw dressing.

Sparkling water with lemon or iced green tea
(optional)

Dinner

4 ounces broiled or barbecued pork tenderloin

⅔ cup cooked instant brown rice

⅔ cup steamed green peas

One steamed artichoke with 2 tablespoons low-
calorie, low-sodium mayonnaise seasoned with
pepper or curry powder

200-Calorie, All-Carb Snack

1 ¼ cups fresh bing cherries and 1 dark chocolate
mini candy bar (Halloween size)

*Cherries are one of the few foods that contain
melatonin, a hormone that helps us sleep.*

Nutritional information without snack: 1,611 calories, 27% fat
(48.4 g total, 13.7 g saturated), 23% protein (91.5 g), 50% carbs (203 g),
28 g fiber, 607 mg calcium, 401 mcg folate, 1,948 mg sodium

Nutritional information with snack: 1,809 calories, 26%
(53 g total, 16 g saturated), 21% protein (95 g), 53% carbs (238 g),
30.5 g fiber, 652 g calcium, 415 mcg folate, 1,988 mg sodium

DAY 11

Breakfast

Orange Sunshine Pancakes: Make these pancakes ahead of time, freeze, then warm in the microwave for an instant breakfast.

Mix ⅓ cup low-fat pancake mix (such as Heart Smart Bisquick), mixed with 2 tablespoons egg substitute, 4 teaspoons toasted wheat germ, 1 tablespoon orange juice concentrate, 1 teaspoon grated orange peel and ¼ cup low-fat milk with DHA. Pour in two equal amounts onto a hot griddle coated with vegetable spray, cook until bubbles on top of each pancake begin to pop, then flip and cook for another two minutes or until done. Top with 2 tablespoons marmalade and ⅓ cup nonfat plain yogurt.

Green tea (optional)

Lunch

Lox, Cream Cheese and Bagel: One whole-wheat bagel with 3 ounces smoked salmon, 1 tablespoon low-fat cream cheese, one slice red onion, 2 tablespoons grated carrot, ¼ red pepper cut into thin strips

1 cup fresh orange juice

Dinner

Pronto Pasta: 1 ½ cup cooked linguini tossed with
1 cup marinara sauce, ½ cup diced onion, two minced
garlic cloves and 1 tablespoon Parmesan cheese.

1 ½ cups steamed broccoli

½ cup lemon sorbet, topped with ¼ cup fresh or
thawed blueberries

200-Calorie, All-Carb Snack

6 cups air-popped popcorn (flavored with chili
powder, garlic powder and/or cumin, if desired)

1 cup sparkling water mixed with ⅓ cup low-calorie
cranberry juice

Nutritional information without snack: 1,599 calories, 17% fat
(29.5 g total, 8.5 g saturated), 17% protein (69 g), 66% carbs (264 g),
27 g fiber, 855 mg calcium, 470 mcg folate, 2,300 mg sodium

Nutritional information with snack: 1,797 calories, 16% (31.5 g total,
8.8 g saturated), 17% protein (75 g), 67% carbs (304 g), 34.5 g fiber,
867 g calcium, 481 mcg folate, 2,304 mg sodium

DAY 12

Breakfast

Berry Ricotta Toast: One slice 100% whole-wheat
toast with 1 tablespoon berry jam and ⅓ cup
part-skim ricotta cheese.

⅔ cup blueberries (pile some on top of the cheese!)

6-ounce glass of grapefruit juice

Coffee with ⅓ cup low-fat milk with DHA

Lunch

BLT: Two slices 100% whole-wheat bread, 1 tablespoon low-fat mayonnaise, one slice Canadian bacon, three thick slices tomato and two lettuce leaves.

Red and Green Salad: 1 cup steamed green beans; 12 cherry tomatoes, halved; 1 teaspoon extra-virgin olive oil; 1 tablespoon balsamic vinegar; 1 minced clove garlic; and salt and pepper to taste.

1 cup low-fat milk with DHA

One tangerine

Dinner

Guiltless Fried Chicken: 4-ounce skinless, boneless chicken breast drizzled with 1 tablespoon low-fat margarine and rolled in ¼ cup bread crumbs seasoned with a pinch of dried thyme and rosemary. Place on cookie sheet coated with vegetable spray, and bake at 400 degrees for 50 minutes.

Sautéed Asparagus: 2 cups asparagus spears sautéed with 2 minced garlic cloves in 1 teaspoon olive oil.

One 6-ounce sweet potato microwaved until soft. Mash with 2 tablespoons low-fat milk, 1 tablespoon dried tart cherries and 1 tablespoon chopped pecans

200-Calorie, All-Carb Snack

Two frozen all-fruit juice bars

Two small oatmeal cookies

Nutritional information without snack: 1,599 calories, 24% fat (42.3 g total, 12 g saturated), 20% protein (80.6 g), 56% carbs (223 g), 31 g fiber, 1,058 mg calcium, 614 mcg folate, 1,608 mg sodium

Nutritional information with snack: 1,796 calories, 23% fat (46.4 g total, 12.8 g saturated), 19% protein (83.6 g), 58% carbs (260 g), 32 g fiber, 1,090 mg calcium, 623 mcg folate, 1,756 mg sodium

DAY 13

Breakfast

Morning Parfait: In a tall glass, layer ⅓ cup low-fat granola; 1 cup low-fat plain yogurt; one medium orange, peeled and chopped; one kiwi, peeled and chopped; and 2 teaspoons dried tart cherries.

Green tea (optional)

Lunch

Chicken Fiesta Salad: 4 cups deep-green lettuce; 1 ounce grated, reduced-fat cheddar cheese; ⅓ cup corn; ⅓ cup canned black beans, drained and rinsed; 2 tablespoons grated carrot; 4 tablespoons diced red onion; 3 ounces roasted or grilled chicken breast; and 2 tablespoons low-fat dressing.

One small 100% whole-wheat roll, topped with 1 teaspoon butter

Water with lemon

Dinner

Juicy, Piled-High Hamburger: One 100% whole-wheat hamburger bun, 2 tablespoons catsup, 1 teaspoon Dijon mustard, 3 ounces extra-lean cooked hamburger (or ground turkey breast meat), two thick tomato slices and three lettuce leaves

One 4-ounce baked potato, topped with 2 tablespoons fat-free sour cream

¾ cup steamed green peas

6 ounces tomato juice

200-Calorie, All-Carb Snack

Two 100% whole-wheat Fig Newtons

6 ounces apricot nectar

Nutritional information without snack: 1,606 calories, 24% fat (42.8 g total, 15.2 g saturated), 25% protein (101.3 g), 51% carbs (206.5 g), 32 g fiber, 1,040 mg calcium, 773 mcg folate, 1,657 mg sodium

Nutritional information with snack: 1,798 calories, 23% fat (45 g total, 15.6 g saturated), 24% protein (108 g), 53% carbs (238 g), 36 g fiber, 1,070 mg calcium, 778 mcg folate, 1,760 mg sodium

DAY 14

Breakfast

1 serving Creamy Oatmeal with Oranges,
Tart Cherries and Nuts*

Low-fat Latte: Coffee and ⅓ cup low-fat milk
with DHA.

Lunch

1 serving of Spinach and Roasted Red Pepper
Frittata*

Tossed Salad: 2 cups deep-green lettuce,
½ cup sliced cucumbers and 2 tablespoons
low-calorie dressing.

Sparkling water with lemon

Dinner

1 serving Ginger Salmon on a Bed of Sautéed
Sesame Spinach*

1 serving Orange Cherry Rice*

1 serving Vanilla Cream Sprinkled with Nuts*

Decaffeinated green tea

200-Calorie, All-Carb Snack

1 Blueberry Spice Muffin*

Nutritional information without snack: 1,695 calories, 38% fat
(72 g total, 21 g saturated), 20% protein (85 g), 42% carbs (178 g),
17 g fiber, 1,162 mg calcium, 444 mcg folate, 1,193 mg sodium

Nutritional information with snack: 1,896 calories, 37% fat
(78 g total, 21.5 g saturated), 19% protein (85 g), 44% carbs (209 g),
20 g fiber, 1,235 g calcium, 456 mcg folate, 1,363 mg sodium

* In Recipes section

RECIPES

BREAKFAST

Plum Nuts Oatmeal

1 ⅔ cups low-fat milk with DHA
⅓ cup pitted dried plums, chopped
2 teaspoons brown sugar
1 tablespoon Splenda
⅛ teaspoon cinnamon
1 cup old-fashioned rolled oats
⅛ teaspoon almond extract
¼ cup low-fat milk with DHA
1 tablespoon sliced almonds

1. In a medium saucepan, bring milk, plums, brown sugar and Splenda to a gentle boil. Add oats and extract. Stir to coat. Return to simmer, lower heat and cook uncovered for 7 minutes or until liquid is absorbed.

2. Portion into two bowls, pour remaining ¼ cup milk over top, and sprinkle with almonds.

Makes 2 servings.

Nutritional information per serving: 365 calories, 16% fat (6.5 g total, 2 g saturated), 67% carbs (61 g), 17% protein (15.5 g), 6 g fiber, 332 mg calcium, 27 mcg folate, 2.6 mg iron, 124 mg sodium

Pumpkin Pie Oatmeal

1 ½ cups soy milk with DHA
½ teaspoon pumpkin spice
1 cup old-fashioned rolled oats
½ cup canned pumpkin
½ teaspoon vanilla extract
1 tablespoon brown sugar
1 tablespoon Splenda
¼ cup low-fat milk with DHA
1 tablespoon chopped almonds
1 teaspoon crystalline ginger bits

1. In a medium saucepan, heat soy milk and pumpkin spice to a gentle boil. Add oats, return to simmer, reduce heat and simmer for 5 minutes.

2. Add pumpkin, vanilla and brown sugar. Cook 1 minute to heat through but not boil.

3. Portion into two bowls, pour milk over top and sprinkle with nuts and crystalline ginger.

Makes 2 servings.

Nutritional information per serving: 302 calories, 20% fat (6.7 g total, < 1 g saturated), 62% carbs (46.8 g), 18% protein (13.6 g), 8.6 g fiber, 389 mg calcium, 25 mcg folate, 3.4 mg iron, 94 mg sodium

Creamy Oatmeal with Oranges, Tart Cherries and Nuts

1 tablespoon chopped walnuts
1 teaspoon maple syrup
1¼ cup low-fat milk with DHA, divided
2 teaspoons orange zest
5 tablespoons chopped tart cherries
2 teaspoons Splenda
⅛ teaspoon nutmeg
dash of salt (optional)
½ cup old-fashioned rolled oats

1. Preheat oven to 350°F.

2. Place nuts in a small bowl and drizzle with maple syrup. Toss and let stand for 10 minutes. Place on tinfoil and bake for 10 minutes or until toasted. Remove and let cool.

3. In a small saucepan, place 1 cup milk, orange zest, cherries, Splenda, nutmeg and salt. Bring to a gentle boil. Add oats, return to boil, reduce heat and simmer for 5 minutes or until almost all liquid is absorbed. Meanwhile, warm remaining ¼ cup milk.

4. Place oats in a bowl, top with remaining milk and toasted pecans. Serve.

Makes 1 serving.

Nutritional information: 507 calories, 18% fat (10 g total, 3 g saturated),
67% carbs (85 g), 15% protein (19 g), 7 g fiber, 439 mg calcium,
36 mcg folate, 3 mg iron, 163 mg sodium

BREADS

Cherry Swirl Strudel Ring with Lemon Glaze

1 packet dry yeast (2 ¼ teaspoons)
2 tablespoons + 1 teaspoon sugar, divided
⅓ cup low-fat milk with DHA
2 teaspoons vanilla extract
1 large egg
2 ¾ cups unbleached all-purpose flour
2 tablespoons Splenda
4 tablespoons butter, cut into small cubes
¼ teaspoon salt
1 egg white
2 teaspoons water

Filling
2 ½ cups dried tart cherries
⅔ cup tart cherry juice
cooking spray

Glaze
¾ cup powdered sugar
1 tablespoon + 1 teaspoon lemon juice
¼ teaspoon lemon extract

1. In a small bowl, place yeast, 1 teaspoon sugar and ¼ cup warm water. Whisk to dissolve yeast, then let sit for 5 minutes. Stir in milk, vanilla and egg. Set aside.

2. In a food processor, place flour, 2 tablespoons sugar, Splenda, butter and salt. Pulse until blended and butter is dispersed throughout flour, giving it a cornmeal texture. Put mixture in medium bowl and add yeast mixture. Stir, then knead until dough forms a ball. Turn dough onto a dry surface (add a bit of flour if dough sticks) and knead lightly for 2 minutes. Dough will feel sticky.

3. Place dough in a medium bowl coated with cooking spray, and turn to coat top. Cover and let rise in a warm place free from drafts until dough has doubled in size. Punch down, knead a few times to evenly disperse temperature, then let rest for 5 minutes.

4. While dough is rising, prepare cherry filling by placing cherries and cherry juice in a blender and blending until liquid (small bits of cherries will be suspended in liquid). Transfer to a medium saucepan and heat over medium heat, stirring frequently until mixture is the consistency of thin jam. Remove from heat and cool. (Cherry mixture will thicken somewhat as it cools.)

5. Place dough on a clean surface and roll into

a 24" x 10" rectangle. Spread cooled cherry mixture evenly over surface, leaving a 1-inch margin along all sides. Starting at one long side, roll dough tightly into a long roll. Pinch seam to seal, using water if necessary.

6. Coat a 12" pizza pan with cooking spray. Place roll on greased pan and bring ends of roll together to form a ring. Pinch ends together to seal, using water if necessary. With scissors, make V-shaped cuts 1 ½" apart, folding V backward to expose cherry filling below. Cover and let rise in a warm place for 30 minutes.

7. Preheat oven to 350°F. Whip egg white and water in a small bowl and brush over top of ring. Bake for 20 to 25 minutes or until golden brown. Cool on rack.

8. Blend powdered sugar, lemon juice and lemon extract in a small bowl and pour evenly over top of cooled ring. Serve at room temperature.

Makes 12 wedges.

Nutritional information per serving: 263 calories, 16% fat (4.7 g total, <1 g saturated), 77% carbs (51 g), 7% protein (4.6 g), 2.2 g fiber, 28 mg calcium, 22 mcg folate, 2 mg iron, 97 mg sodium

Blueberry Spice Muffins

2 cups + 1 tablespoon whole-wheat flour, divided
½ cup + 5 teaspoons sugar, divided
¼ cup Splenda
1 tablespoon baking powder
¼ teaspoon salt
½ teaspoon ground cinnamon
⅛ teaspoon ground cloves
⅛ teaspoon ground nutmeg
1 ½ cups fresh or thawed blueberries
⅓ cup canola oil
8 ounces fat-free cream cheese
½ cup soy milk with DHA
2 eggs
1 teaspoon vanilla extract

1. Heat oven to 425°F. Coat 12-cup muffin pan with cooking spray.

2. In a large bowl, thoroughly mix 2 cups flour, ½ cup sugar, Splenda, baking powder, salt, cinnamon, cloves and nutmeg. Set aside.

3. In a small bowl, toss blueberries with 1 tablespoon flour. Set aside.

4. In a medium bowl, blend oil and cream cheese with an electric mixer until creamed. Add soy milk, eggs, and vanilla slowly, and blend until thoroughly creamed. Add to flour mixture and stir just until moistened. Gently mix in blueberries.

5. Spoon batter evenly into muffin cups. Sprinkle with remaining sugar. Bake until muffins spring back, or approximately 15 minutes. Remove from pan and cool on wire rack.

Makes 12 muffins.

Nutritional information per muffin: 200 calories, 31% fat (6.9 g total, <1 g saturated), 57% carbs (28.5 g), 12% protein (6 g), 3 g fiber, 74 mg calcium, 12 mcg folate, 1 mg iron, 170 mg sodium

SALADS & SOUP

Spiced-up Tofu, Orange and Avocado Salad

Tofu
¼ cup hoisin sauce
2 tablespoons low-sodium soy sauce
5 teaspoons minced fresh ginger
pinch of red pepper flakes
1 large clove garlic, minced
1 tablespoon olive oil
1 package extra-firm tofu, drained and patted dry

Dressing
2 tablespoons freshly squeezed orange juice
2 tablespoons rice wine vinegar
1 tablespoon sesame oil
½ teaspoon grated orange peel
salt and pepper to taste

Salad
2 bags spring lettuce leaves
⅔ cup thinly sliced red onion
3 navel oranges, peeled, pith removed,
    and cut into thin rounds
1 large avocado, peeled and sliced thin

1. In a small bowl, blend hoisin sauce, soy sauce, ginger, pepper flakes and garlic. Set aside.

2. Place olive oil in a large nonstick frying pan and heat on medium heat until hot. Add tofu cubes and sauté until golden brown on all sides, approximately 10 minutes.

3. Add hoisin mix, toss to coat tofu and reduce heat to low. Simmer until sauce evaporates, turning tofu occasionally, approximately 10 minutes. Remove from heat.

4. In a small bowl, blend orange juice, vinegar, oil, orange peel and salt and pepper. Set aside.

5. Place lettuce and onion in a large bowl. Toss with dressing. Divide between four plates and top with tofu, oranges and avocado slices.

Makes 6 servings.

Nutritional information per serving: 245 calories, 51% fat (13.8 g total, 2 g saturated), 30% carbs (18.4 g), 19% protein (11.6 g), 5 g fiber, 217 mg calcium, 193 mcg folate, 8.2 mg iron, 468 mg sodium

Beets 'n' Blue Cheese Salad

⅓ cup freshly squeezed lemon juice

2 tablespoons sugar

1 tablespoon Splenda

3 tablespoons finely chopped red onion

1 tablespoon extra-virgin olive oil

salt to taste

1 pound beets

12 cups mixed salad greens

3 tablespoons cashews

3 tablespoons crumbled blue cheese

1. Preheat oven to 350°F.

2. Mix first six ingredients together, stir and refrigerate.

3. Remove root and stems from beets, wash and place in baking dish with ¼ inch water. Cover and bake until barely tender. Time will vary from 35 minutes to 1 hour. Remove when tender. Cool. Rub off skins and cut into chunks. Set aside.

4. Place greens in large bowl or platter. Top with beets, cashews and blue cheese. Drizzle dressing over top and serve.

Makes 8 large servings.

Nutritional information per serving: 100 calories, 37% fat (4 g total, 1 g saturated), 50% carbs (12.5 g), 13% protein (3.3 g), 3 g fiber, 74 mg calcium, 146 mcg folate, 1.8 mg iron, 129 mg sodium

Mango, Cranberries and Avocado Toss

8 cups leaf lettuce
3 tablespoons orange juice
1 tablespoon rice wine vinegar
½ teaspoon dry mustard
1 teaspoon coriander seeds, coarsely cracked
1 tablespoon honey
1 tablespoon olive oil
salt and pepper to taste
½ cup diced red onion
2 ripe avocados, peeled, seeded and sliced thin
1 ripe mango, peeled, seeded and chopped
1 ⅓ cups dried cranberries

1. Divide lettuce evenly onto four salad plates. Set aside.

2. In a small bowl, whisk together orange juice, vinegar, mustard, coriander seeds, honey, olive oil, and salt and pepper. Set aside.

3. Layer evenly atop each of the lettuce heaps the diced red onion, the avocado slices, the mango chunks and the cranberries. Drizzle the dressing over the top and serve immediately.

Makes 4 servings.

Nutritional information per serving: 333 calories, 38% fat (14.1 g total, 2.2 g saturated), 5% protein (4.2 g), 57% carbs (47.5 g), 7 g fiber, 94 mg calcium, 184 mcg folate, 3.7 mg iron, 46 mg sodium

Sage-Infused Roasted Butternut Squash Soup

1 butternut squash, peeled, seeded and cubed
     (approximately 3 ½ pounds)
4 carrots, peeled and sliced
2 baking potatoes, peeled and cubed
2 cups chopped onions
1 32-ounce carton low-sodium chicken broth
2 ½ cups soy milk with DHA
2 teaspoons powdered sage
3 tablespoons lemon juice
1 tablespoon brown sugar
salt to taste
1 7-ounce jar roasted red peppers
pinch of cayenne

1. Heat oven to 400°F. Coat baking sheet with cooking spray.

2. Place squash on baking sheet. Spray with cooking spray and roast until tender, stirring occasionally, approximately 30 minutes. Remove and set aside.

3. While squash is roasting, steam carrots for 5 minutes. Add potatoes and onions and continue to steam until tender.

4. In a blender or food processor, puree squash and vegetables in small batches until smooth, adding chicken broth as needed to blend.

5. Place vegetable puree in a large saucepan, along with any remaining broth. Add soy milk, sage, lemon juice, sugar and salt. Stir over medium heat to blend seasonings.

6. Blend roasted red peppers with cayenne in a blender until smooth. Drizzle across each bowl of soup, then run a fork through the drizzle.

Makes 8 servings.

Nutritional information per serving: 254 calories, 6% fat (1.7 g total, 0 g saturated), 81% carbs (51 g), 13% protein (8.3 g), 10 g fiber, 239 mg calcium, 65 mcg folate, 3 mg iron, 420 mg sodium

LUNCHES & SNACKS

Minty Rice, Orange and Pomegranate Bowl

4 cups cooked brown rice

½ teaspoon salt

1 heaping tablespoon finely grated orange peel

⅓ cup fresh orange juice
(or juice of one large orange)

½ cup champagne vinegar

1 tablespoon extra-virgin olive oil

¼ teaspoon freshly ground black pepper

2 ¼ cups orange sections (approximately
3 oranges, peeled, sectioned, and then cut
crosswise into halves)

⅔ cup pomegranate seeds (use dried cranberries
    when pomegranates are out of season)
2 tablespoons chopped mint
¼ cup toasted slivered almonds

1. Place rice in a medium bowl.

2. In a small bowl, whisk orange peel, orange juice,
vinegar, oil, salt and pepper. Pour over rice and
blend well.

3. Add orange sections, pomegranate seeds, mint
and almonds. Toss gently until well mixed.

Makes approximately six 1-cup servings.

Nutritional information per cup: 280 calories, 16% fat
(4.9 g total, <1 g saturated), 76% carbs (53 g), 8% protein (5.6 g),
3.6 g fiber, 57 mg calcium, 33 mcg folate, 2 mg iron, 181 mg sodium

Spicy Salmon Tacos

juice of one large lemon
1 teaspoon chili powder
1 teaspoon paprika
salt to taste
1 ¼ pounds wild salmon fillet
⅔ cup commercial salsa
1 cup chopped tomato
2 tablespoons minced red onion
3 tablespoons chopped cilantro
4 cups shredded cabbage

⅔ cup canned black beans, drained and rinsed

½ cup fat-free sour cream

1 large avocado, peeled and cubed (doused with
    lemon juice to prevent browning)

15 organic corn tortillas

1. In a shallow pan, mix lemon juice, chili powder, paprika and salt. Place salmon in pan, coat both sides, cover and refrigerate for up to 12 hours.

2. Heat broiler. Line baking sheet with tinfoil and spray with cooking spray.

3. In a medium bowl, mix salsa, tomatoes, onion and cilantro. Set aside.

4. Broil fish until cooked through, turning fish halfway through cooking time. Broil for 10 minutes for every inch of thickness. (If fish is less than ½ an inch thick, don't turn.) Remove from oven, cool slightly and break into chunks. Set aside.

5. Place cabbage, black beans, sour cream and avocado in separate serving bowls. Set aside.

6. Heat a nonstick griddle on medium-high heat. Place tortillas on griddle and warm, turning once.

7. Fill each tortilla with a small helping of fish, the salsa mixture, cabbage, black beans, avocado and sour cream. Ingredients will keep in refrigerator for up to two days.

Makes 15 tacos.

Nutritional information per taco: 180 calories, 33% fat
(6.6 g total, 1.4 g saturated), 43% carbs (19.4 g),
24% protein (10.8 g), 3 g fiber, 75 mg calcium, 46 mcg folate,
1.2 mg iron, 119 mg sodium

Wasabi 'n' Ginger Salmon Sandwiches

¼ cup fat-free mayonnaise
¼ to ½ teaspoon wasabi paste
8 thin (1-ounce) slices from a loaf of bakery
    French or sourdough bread
8 ounces cooked salmon, divided into
    four equal servings
4 thin slices red onion, separated
16 thin slices red pepper
4 tablespoons pickled sliced ginger
1 cup baby spinach or baby wild greens

1. In a small bowl, thoroughly mix mayonnaise
and wasabi paste. Start with ¼ teaspoon of the
paste and add more to suit your taste. Set aside.

2. Place four slices of bread on a flat surface and
spread each with 1 tablespoon of the mayonnaise-
wasabi mixture. Top with 2 ounces salmon, one
slice onion spread evenly over salmon, four slices
red pepper, 1 tablespoon pickled ginger, and
¼ cup greens. Top with remaining four slices
of bread.

Makes 4 sandwiches.

Nutritional information per sandwich: 302 calories, 24% fat
(8 g total, 1.5 g saturated), 46% carbs (35.5 g), 29% protein (22 g),
2.4 g fiber, 66 mg calcium, 53 mcg folate, 2.3 mg iron, 564 mg sodium

SIDE DISHES

Cherry & Apple Stuffed Acorn Squash

2 acorn squash, halved and seeded
salt
1 ½ cups dried tart cherries
⅓ cup tart cherry juice
1 ½ cups Granny Smith apples, peeled, seeded
   and diced
1 tablespoon butter
½ teaspoon rum extract (optional)
4 tablespoons chopped pecans
4 teaspoons dark honey

1. Preheat oven to 350°F. Coat a baking sheet with
cooking spray.

2. Lightly salt the 4 acorn squash halves, place cut
side down on baking sheet and bake for 25 minutes.
Remove from oven.

3. While squash is baking, place cherries and juice
in a medium saucepan. Bring to a boil, reduce heat

and simmer until cherries soak up liquid. Add apples and butter. Continue to simmer for 5 minutes, or until apples are heated through but not soft. (For an extra-rich taste, add ½ teaspoon of rum extract to the cherry-apple mixture after removing from stove.)

4. Divide cherry filling into four equal portions and fill each of the four squash halves. Sprinkle with a tablespoon of pecans and drizzle with 1 teaspoon of honey. Return to oven and bake for an additional 15 minutes. Serve warm.

Makes 4 servings.

Nutritional information per serving: 367 calories, 19% fat (7.7 g total, 2 g saturated), 77% carbs (70.6 g), 4% protein (3.7 g), 12 g fiber, 117 mg calcium, 44 mcg folate, 3.6 mg iron, 181 mg sodium

---

Orange-Glazed Roasted Brussels Sprouts and Cauliflower

1 pound Brussels sprouts, trimmed
1 head cauliflower, trimmed and cut into florets
¼ cup red onion, diced
4 cloves garlic, minced
2 tablespoons orange peel, minced
¼ cup olive oil
⅛ teaspoon red pepper flakes
salt to taste

⅓ cup orange juice
1 tablespoon orange juice concentrate
orange slices

1. Heat oven to 450°F. Coat baking sheet with cooking spray.

2. Combine Brussels sprouts, cauliflower, onion, garlic, orange peel, oil, red pepper flakes and salt in a large bowl. Toss well. Spread on baking sheet and roast for 15 minutes or until slightly golden but still firm. Stir once during roasting. Remove from oven.

3. In a small bowl, blend orange juice with orange juice concentrate. Pour over vegetables and return to oven. Roast for another 10 minutes or until vegetables are firm but done and juice has evaporated. Garnish with orange slices.

Makes 8 servings.

Nutritional information per serving: 107 calories, 55% fat (6.5 g total, 1 g saturated), 35% carbs (9.4 g), 10% protein (2.7 g), 4 g fiber, 40 mg calcium, 64 mcg folate, 1 mg iron, 26 mg sodium

Mashed Roasted Sweet Potatoes with a Taste of Honey

3 pounds sweet potatoes, peeled and cut
    into 1" cubes
3 tablespoons honey

2 tablespoons butter, melted
⅓ cup fat-free sour cream
pinch of red pepper flakes
salt to taste
3 tablespoons chopped pistachios

1. Preheat oven to 400°F. Coat baking sheet with cooking spray.

2. Place potatoes in a single layer on cookie sheet. Lightly spray with cooking spray. Bake for approximately 40 minutes or until tender, stirring occasionally.

3. In a large bowl, place cooked potatoes and honey, butter, sour cream, red pepper flakes and salt. Beat with a mixer until smooth and creamy. Sprinkle with pistachios and serve.

Makes 8 servings.

Nutritional information per serving: 247 calories, 16% fat (4.4 g total, 2 g saturated), 77% carbs (47.5 g), 7% protein (4.3 g), 5.4 g fiber, 53 mg calcium, 41 mcg folate, 1 mg iron, 53 mg sodium

Nutty Green Tea Rice

tea leaves from four bags of green tea
1 cup white rice
2 tablespoons Splenda
2 tablespoons champagne or
    white wine vinegar

salt to taste

1 tablespoon slivered almonds

1. Combine tea leaves, rice and 2 cups water in a medium saucepan over high heat. Bring to a boil, reduce heat and simmer until all water is absorbed, about 20 minutes.

2. In a small bowl, combine Splenda, vinegar and salt. Whisk together until blended.

3. Pour vinegar mixture into rice and blend. Divide into four servings and sprinkle with almonds.

Makes 4 servings.

Nutritional information per serving: 179 calories, 6% fat (1.2 g total, 0 g saturated), 86% carbs (38.5 g), 8% protein (3.6 g), 0.6 g fiber, 17 mg calcium, 4 mcg folate, 2 mg iron, 2.6 mg sodium

Orange Cherry Rice

1 large or 2 medium oranges

3 cups brown basmati rice

⅓ cup slivered almonds

1 tablespoon sugar

⅔ cup dried tart cherries

salt to taste

1. Grate or zest the orange peel and set aside the zest. Remove the white pith and liquify the orange(s) in a blender.

2. Place orange zest in saucepan with 2 cups water and bring to boil. Reduce heat and simmer for 10 minutes. Remove peel and set aside. Save water.

3. Place orange water in a medium saucepan with the liquified orange, and add additional water to match directions for cooking rice on package (approximately 6 cups). Salt to taste, bring to boil, add rice, return to boil, then lower heat and simmer covered until liquid is absorbed and rice is cooked.

4. While rice is cooking, place almonds in a nonstick frying pan over medium heat and toast, stirring frequently, until golden brown, approximately 7 minutes. Remove from pan and set aside.

5. Place orange zest, sugar, and ½ cup water in a nonstick frying pan. Bring to boil, reduce heat and simmer until liquid has evaporated, stirring frequently. Remove from pan and set aside.

6. Place cherries in a nonstick frying pan with ½ cup water, bring to boil, reduce heat and simmer until liquid has evaporated. Remove from pan and set aside.

7. When rice is cooked, add orange peel, cherries and almonds. Toss to mix thoroughly.

Makes 8 cups, or 12 servings.

Nutritional information per serving: 227 calories, 11% fat (2.8 g total, 0 g saturated), 80% carbs (45 g), 8% protein (4.5 g), 3g fiber, 29 mg calcium, 16 mcg folate, 1 mg iron, 5 mg sodium

DINNER

Seared Salmon with Mango-Mint Salsa

Salsa

1 12-ounce mango, peeled, seeded and chopped
(produces about 1 ½ cups)
⅓ cup diced red pepper
¼ cup diced red onion
1 scant tablespoon chopped jalapeño
(more if you like very spicy foods!)
2 tablespoons chopped fresh mint
salt and pepper to taste
1 tablespoon freshly squeezed lime juice

Salmon

1 pound salmon fillet, about 1 inch thick
¼ cup freshly squeezed lemon juice
(about the juice of one lemon)
⅛ teaspoon paprika
salt and pepper to taste
1 teaspoon olive oil

1. To make salsa, blend all ingredients (mango
through lime juice) in a small bowl. Cover and
refrigerate for up to two hours. (Flavors blend
best when salsa sits for an hour or more.)

2. Place salmon fillet in a large shallow baking dish.
In a small bowl, mix lemon juice, paprika, salt and

pepper. Pour over salmon, covering both sides. Marinate for up to one hour. Drain fillet just before cooking.

3. Pour olive oil into a large nonstick skillet and heat over medium-high heat. Place fillet in pan (you may need to cut in half to fit) and sear four to six minutes per side, depending on thickness of fish and degree of desired doneness.

4. Place fillet on platter and top with salsa.

Makes 4 servings.

Nutritional information per serving: 280 calories, 42% fat (13.1 g total, 3 g saturated), 25% carbs (17.5 g), 33% protein (23.1 g), 2.2 g fiber, 41 mg calcium, 59 mcg folate, 67 mg sodium

Ginger Salmon on a Bed of Sautéed Sesame Spinach

⅓ cup bottled hoisin sauce

2 ½ tablespoons peeled and minced fresh ginger

1 teaspoon brown sugar

2 teaspoons canned chipotle peppers, diced

¼ cup chopped fresh cilantro

1 pound wild salmon fillet

3 tablespoons freshly squeezed lemon juice

1 tablespoon olive oil

1 clove garlic, minced

pinch of crushed red pepper flakes (optional)

2 10-ounce boxes frozen chopped spinach, thawed
salt to taste
1 tablespoon sesame seeds

1. Preheat broiler. Line baking sheet with tinfoil.

2. In a small bowl, stir together hoisin sauce, ginger, brown sugar, chipotle and cilantro.

3. Rinse and dry salmon. Rub with lemon juice, then brush both sides with sauce mixture, place on foil-lined baking sheet, cover and refrigerate while preparing spinach.

4. In a large nonstick frying pan, heat olive oil over medium heat. Add garlic and sauté, stirring continuously so as not to burn for two minutes. (If you like a little "zing," then add crushed red pepper flakes during last 30 seconds of sautéing the garlic.) Add spinach and sauté until heated through. Remove from heat and keep warm. (Or prepare spinach while salmon is in broiler.)

5. Broil salmon until opaque in center, basting occasionally with remaining sauce (approximately six minutes, depending on thickness of fish).

6. Place spinach on serving platter, sprinkle with sesame seeds and top with salmon.

Makes 4 servings.

Nutritional information per serving: 289 calories, 53% fat (17 g total, 3.6 g saturated), 11% carbs (8 g), 36% protein (26 g), 2 g fiber, 115 mg calcium, 126 mcg folate, 2.7 mg iron, 292 mg sodium

Linguini à la Pomodori

salt

½ pound whole-grain linguini

1 pound fresh Roma tomatoes, chopped
    (approximately 2 cups)

⅓ cup sun-dried tomatoes, chopped

¾ cup yellow bell peppers, washed, seeded and
    cut into thin 2"-long slivers

½ cup packed fresh basil leaves, chopped

2 cloves garlic, minced

3 tablespoons fresh Italian parsley, minced

2 ounces gorgonzola cheese, crumbled

2 ounces fat-free feta cheese, crumbled

1. Bring a large pot of salted water to a boil,
add linguini and cook according to directions
on package (approximately 10 to 12 minutes).
Remove from heat and drain.

2. Meanwhile, in a large bowl, toss the tomatoes,
peppers, basil, garlic, parsley, gorgonzola and feta
cheese. Add pasta and toss until gorgonzola begins
to melt.

Makes 4 generous servings, approximately
1 ½ cups each.

Nutritional information per serving: 256 calories, 19% fat (5.4 g total,
3 g saturated), 60% carbs (38.4 g), 21% protein (13.4 g), 7 g fiber,
168 mg calcium, 42 mcg folate, 2.6 mg iron, 590 mg sodium

Curried Butternut Squash with Chutney and Rice

4 cups fat-free chicken broth, divided
1 ½ cups basmati brown rice
1 tablespoon extra-virgin olive oil
1 large onion, peeled and cut into ½" rings
3 cloves garlic, minced
5 cups butternut squash, peeled and cut into
   1" cubes (approximately 12 ounces)
1 tablespoon curry powder
salt to taste
½ cup fat-free half & half
pinch of red pepper flakes
⅓ cup chopped peanuts
½ cup bottled chutney

1. Bring 3 cups chicken broth to a boil in medium saucepan over high heat. Add rice, reduce heat and simmer until done, approximately 35 minutes.

2. Heat oil in large nonstick skillet over medium heat. Add onions and sauté for five minutes until softened. Add garlic, squash, curry and salt. Toss to coat. Add 1 cup broth and cover. Cook until squash is semisoft but still firm and liquid is almost evaporated.

3. Add half & half and red pepper flakes. Cook until sauce thickens, stirring occasionally. Remove from heat.

4. Portion rice and top with butternut squash mixture into serving bowls. Top with peanuts and chutney.

Makes 6 servings.

Nutritional information per serving: 392 calories, 20% fat (8.7 g total, 1.5 g saturated), 68% carbs (66.6 g), 12% protein (11.8 g), 8.2 g fiber, 120 mg calcium, 64 mcg folate, 2.6 mg iron, 579 mg sodium

---

Spinach and Roasted Red Pepper Frittata

3 red peppers, stemmed, seeded and cut
    into quarters
1 cup fat-free half & half
1 ½ cup egg substitute
1 cup low-fat ricotta cheese
¾ cup grated reduced-fat cheese with DHA
⅓ cup low-fat grated Parmesan cheese
1 tablespoon olive oil
⅓ cup onion, chopped
4 cloves garlic, minced
4 6-ounce bags baby spinach
salt and pepper to taste

1. Preheat oven to 400°F. Coat baking sheet with cooking spray. Coat 13" x 9" x 2" baking dish with cooking spray.

2. Place peppers on cookie sheet, spray with cooking spray and roast until tender but not soft,

approximately 20 minutes. Cool and cut into
¼" strips.

3. In a large bowl, blend half & half, egg substitute
and cheeses. Set aside.

4. Heat olive oil in a large nonstick pan, add onion
and garlic and sauté for five minutes. Add one bag
of spinach and heat until spinach is dark green
and wilted, stirring constantly, approximately two
minutes. Remove onion-spinach mixture and place
in bowl. Add second bag of spinach and repeat,
stirring, for two minutes. Add spinach to onion-
spinach mixture. Repeat until all four bags of
spinach have been sautéed.

5. Stir spinach and two-thirds of the roasted red
pepper strips into egg mixture (reserve one-third of
peppers for topping). (Can be prepared to this point
up to one day in advance. Cover and refrigerate
until ready to bake.)

6. Pour spinach-egg mixture into baking dish.
Bake until knife inserted into center comes out
clean, approximately one hour. Remove from oven,
arrange remaining pepper strips over top and serve.

Makes 8 servings.

Nutritional information per serving: 238 calories, 37% fat (9.8 g total,
3 g saturated), 28% carbs (16.6g), 35% protein (21 g), 3.7 g fiber,
407 mg calcium, 243 mcg folate, 5 mg iron, 331 mg sodium

BEVERAGES

Pineapple Coconut Smoothie

1 cup cubed fresh pineapple
⅓ cup soy milk with DHA
6 ounce container of low-fat piña colada yogurt
¼ + ⅛ teaspoon coconut extract
½ cup crushed ice
lime zest for garnish

Place pineapple, soy milk, yogurt and coconut extract in a blender and whip until smooth. Add ice and whip briefly to mix. Pour into a tall glass and garnish with lime zest.

Makes 1 serving.

Nutritional information: 250 calories, 13% fat (3.6 g total, 1 g saturated), 70% carbs (43.8 g), 17% protein (10.6 g), 3 g fiber, 434 mg calcium, 34 mcg folate, 1 mg iron, 145 mg sodium

Mango-Pineapple Crush

1 ripe mango, peeled, pitted and cubed
    (approximately 1 cup)
½ cup pineapple chunks, preferably fresh
one 6-ounce container low-fat lemon-flavored
    yogurt

2 tablespoons freshly squeezed lemon juice
1 ½ teaspoons rum extract
crushed ice

Place all ingredients, except ice, in a blender and blend on high until smooth. Add ice and blend for another 15 seconds. Pour into glass.

Makes 1 serving.

Nutritional information: 345 calories, 8% fat (3.1 g total, 1.5 g saturated), 81% carbs (70 g), 11% protein (9.5 g), 5.2 g fiber, 319 mg calcium, 69 mcg folate, 0.7 mg iron, 117 mg sodium

Orange Cranberry Fizz

25 fresh cranberries
1 ½ cups ice, crushed
1 cup soy milk with DHA
2 tablespoons Splenda
1 6-ounce can of orange juice concentrate
1 cup sparkling water
5 teaspoons cranberry-orange relish

1. Place fresh cranberries in ice-cube trays, fill with water and freeze.

2. Place remaining ice, soy milk, Splenda and orange juice concentrate in blender. Cover and blend on high speed 30 seconds or until smooth. Turn off blender and pour in sparkling water. Stir.

3. Place two cranberry ice cubes in each of five 6-ounce glasses. Pour in frosty mix and top with a teaspoon of relish. Serve immediately.

Makes five 8-ounce servings.

Nutritional information per serving: 80 calories, 6% fat (0 g total, 0 g saturated), 84% carbs (16.8 g), 10% protein (2 g), 1 g fiber, 92 mg calcium, 53 mcg folate, 0 mg iron, 22 mg sodium

DESSERTS

Poached Pears in Chocolate Lavender Sauce

4 large firm pears (Anjou, Bosc or Bartlett)
¾ cup honey, divided
zest of one orange
1 tablespoon culinary lavender
2 tablespoons cocoa powder
lavender sprigs for garnish (optional)

1. Peel pears and slice bottom so pears will stand up (leave stem at top). Place in a microwave dish and spoon 1 tablespoon honey over each pear. Cover dish and microwave on high for 10 to 12 minutes, or until pears are tender but not too soft. Set aside.

2. Meanwhile, place 1 cup water and ½ cup honey in a saucepan over medium-high heat, bring to boil, reduce heat and simmer until liquid has reduced to half. Add zest, lavender and cocoa and continue to simmer for five minutes, stirring frequently. Strain liquid to remove zest and lavender. Liquid should be a thin syrup.

3. Place pears on individual plates and drizzle chocolate lavender sauce over top, so that it runs down sides and pools at the bottom. Garnish with lavender sprigs and serve.

Makes 4 servings.

Nutritional information per serving: 325 calories, 3% fat (1.1 g total, 0 g saturated), 95% carbs (77 g), 2% protein (1.6 g), 7.2 g fiber, 35 mg calcium, 18 mcg folate, 1.2 mg iron, 3 mg sodium

Vanilla Cream Sprinkled with Nuts

3 tablespoons sugar
3 tablespoons Splenda
2 cups low-fat milk with DHA
dash of salt
1 large egg, beaten
1 teaspoon vanilla extract
3 tablespoons toasted nuts, chopped
dash of nutmeg

1. In a blender, combine sugar, Splenda, milk and salt. Blend. Pour into a medium saucepan and heat over medium-high heat until mixture begins to simmer. Reduce heat and stir for five minutes with mixture at a gentle boil.

2. Place egg in medium bowl. Gradually add heated milk mixture, stirring constantly. Return egg-milk mixture to saucepan and cook over medium heat for three minutes or until mixture thickens, stirring constantly. Remove from heat. Add vanilla to mixture and blend. Pour into a medium bowl and cover surface with plastic wrap.

3. To serve, portion ¼ of mixture into four small bowls. Sprinkle with toasted nuts and nutmeg.

Makes 4 servings.

Nutritional information per serving: 144 calories, 34% fat (5.4 g total, 1.6 g saturated), 47% carbs (16.9 g), 19% protein (6.8 g), 0.7 g fiber, 164 mg calcium, 16 mcg folate, 0.7 mg iron, 78 mg sodium

Chewy, Crunchy, Super Chocolatey Clusters

8 ounces semisweet chocolate with at least
    60% cocoa powder
1 tablespoon cocoa powder
¾ cup dried tart cherries
¾ cup chopped almonds

1. Cover baking sheet with tinfoil and coat with vegetable spray.

2. Place chocolate and cocoa powder in a medium saucepan. Heat over medium-low heat, stirring occasionally, until all chocolate has melted.

3. Stir in cherries and almonds. Immediately drop in small clusters onto baking sheet. Refrigerate until chocolate hardens, approximately 30 minutes.

Makes 30 one-cluster servings.

Nutritional information per cluster: 70 calories, 55% fat (4.3 g total, 1.9 g saturated), 38% carbs (6.7 g), 7% protein (1.2 g), 1 g fiber, 16 mg calcium, 3 mcg folate, 0.6 mg iron, 1 mg sodium

Spiced Panna Cotta with Strawberry-Shiraz Compote

Panna Cotta

1 packet unflavored gelatin (approximately
    2 ½ teaspoons)
¼ cup water
1 ¼ cup evaporated nonfat milk
¼ cup Splenda
2 cups plain nonfat yogurt
¼ teaspoon cardamom
1 teaspoon vanilla extract

Compote

3 cups fresh or thawed frozen strawberries, chopped
⅓ cup Shiraz
1 tablespoon cornstarch
2 tablespoons sugar
2 tablespoons Splenda
lemon zest (optional)

1. Mix gelatin and ¼ cup water in a small bowl and set aside.

2. In a medium saucepan, bring milk, sugar and Splenda to a boil, stirring constantly. Remove from heat and stir in gelatin mixture. Whisk until thoroughly blended. Add yogurt, cardamom and vanilla. Stir until well mixed. Divide into six custard cups and cover and refrigerate overnight.

3. Place berries in a medium saucepan over medium-high heat. Mix wine and cornstarch in a small glass. Add to berries, along with sugar and Splenda. Bring to a boil, stirring constantly. Remove from heat when sauce thickens and turns clear. Cool completely.

4. Run thin sharp knife around the edges of the custard cups or set each ramekin in hot water for one minute to loosen. Place plate on top of ramekin and invert to allow panna cotta to settle onto plate. Top with compote, and sprinkle with lemon zest if desired.

Makes 6 servings.

Nutritional information per serving: 178 calories, 4% fat (<1 g total, 0 g saturated), 70% carbs (31 g), 23% protein (10 g), 2 g fiber, 328 mg calcium, 28 mcg folate, .6 mg iron, 127 mg sodium

Soy Good Pumpkin Pie

1 commercial pie crust (frozen, made according
    to directions, or refrigerated)
1 15-ounce can pumpkin puree
½ cup brown sugar
¼ cup Splenda
1 ⅓ cups soy milk with DHA
1 tablespoon cornstarch
½ teaspoon salt
¾ teaspoon ground cinnamon
½ teaspoon ground ginger
¼ teaspoon ground cloves
¼ teaspoon freshly ground nutmeg
¾ teaspoon vanilla extract
½ cup liquid egg substitute
1 egg, separated into yolk and white
8 tablespoons fat-free whipped topping

1. Preheat oven to 425°F.

2. Roll pie crust to fit a deep-dish pie pan. Press pie crust gently into pan and trim dough to 1 inch from edge of pie pan. Fold under and pinch to form fluted edges. Set aside.

3. In a large bowl, blend pumpkin, sugar, Splenda, soy milk, cornstarch, spices and vanilla.

4. Place egg substitute and 1 egg yolk in a small bowl and beat. Add to pumpkin mixture and blend thoroughly.

5. Beat remaining egg white with electric mixer until soft peaks form. Fold into pumpkin mixture until no white streaks remain. Pour pumpkin filling into pie pan and bake at 425°F for 15 minutes, reduce heat, and bake at 350°F for 50 minutes, or until a toothpick inserted into middle of pie comes out clean. Remove from oven and cool for at least two hours. Top each slice with 1 tablespoon whipped topping.

Makes 8 servings.

Nutritional information per serving: 191 calories, 41% fat (8.7 g total, 3.3 g saturated), 48% carbs (23 g), 11% protein (5 g), 2 g fiber, 93 mg calcium, 12 mcg folate, 1.3 mg iron, 300 mg sodium

APPENDIX

100+ PRODUCTS THAT MEET MOST OF THE REAL-FOOD GUIDELINES

Meats/Protein
Diestel Turkey Breast, Honey Roasted
Healthy Ones 97% Fat-Free Deli Thin Sliced Oven-Roasted
    Turkey Breast
Heidi's Hens Organic Turkey Breast
Hormel 97% Fat-Free, 100% Natural, Carved
    Chicken Breast Grilled
Hormel Natural Choice Smoked Deli Turkey
Jennie-O Extra-Lean Turkey Bacon
Lightlife Smart Bacon (soy)
Mori Nu Silken Lite Tofu
Organic Prairie Hardwood Smoked Ham
Oscar Mayer 98% Fat-Free Wieners (high in sodium)
Tyson 100% All-Natural Boneless Skinless Chicken Breasts

Cereals
Arrowhead Mills Shredded Wheat
Arrowhead Mills Rice & Shine Hot Cereal
Barbara's Bakery Shredded Oats
Bob's Red Mill Organic Whole-Grain Rolled Oats
Bob's Red Mill Kamut Cereal
Cascadian Farm Organic Hearty Morning Cereal
Ezekiel 4:9 Golden Flax Sprouted Whole-Grain Cereal
Kashi Autumn Wheat or 7 Whole-Grain Nuggets Cereal
Nature's Path Organic Flax Plus Raisin Bran Cereal
Quaker Simple Harvest Instant Multigrain Hot Cereal

Breads
Arnold Whole-Grain Classics 100% Whole-Wheat
    (available east of the Mississippi)

Earth Grains Extra-Fiber 100% Whole-Wheat
Oroweat Country Oven 100% Whole-Wheat Bread
Oroweat 100% Whole-Wheat Hamburger Buns
Querro Whole-What Flour Tortillas
Rubschlager 100% Whole Wheat
Thomas Squares Bagelbread 100% Whole Wheat

Grains
Barilla Whole-Grain Pasta
Bionaturae Organic 100% Whole-Wheat Pasta
Heartland Whole-Grain Pasta
Kashi 7 Whole-Grain Pilaf
Reese Quick Cooking Minnesota Wild Rice
Van's All-Natural Gourmet Frozen Waffles
Vita Spelt Whole-Grain Rotini

Canned Goods
Amy's Vegetarian Organic Refried Beans
Barilla Mushroom Garlic Spaghetti Sauce
Bush's Best Black Beans or Garbanzo Beans
    (a bit high in sodium)
Campbell's Healthy Request soups
Classico Signature Recipe's Spicy Red Pepper Pasta Sauce
Del Monte Fresh-Cut Sweet Peas
Del Monte Fresh-Cut Leaf Spinach
Eden Organic Butter Beans
Farmer's Market Organic Sweet Potato Puree
    or Butternut Squash
Health Valley Organic Vegetable Soup
Mt. Olive Reduced-Sodium Kosher Baby Dills
    and Kosher Dill Strips
Napoleon Pimiento Stuffed Olives
Pace salsas
Progresso 50% Less Sodium Chicken Gumbo Soup
S&W Premium Kidney Beans
S&W Cut Green Beans
Swanson's 50% Reduced-Sodium broths

Frozen Entrées
Chicken Entrées: most Healthy Choices, Weight Watchers, or Lean Cuisine Café or Spa Cuisine Classic entrées are fine, but high in sodium
A.C. La Rocco Cheese & Garlic Pizza
Gardenburger: The Original Veggie Burger
Kashi Black Bean Mano, Sweet & Sour Chicken, and Chicken Pasta Pomodoro entrées
Lean Cuisine Salmon with Basil entrée
Lean Cuisine Spa Lemongrass Chicken
Organic Bistro Wild Salmon with Rosemary Orange Glaze
Organic Fresh Fingers Black Bean Burgers
Organic Fresh Fingers Asian-Style Brown Rice
Weight Watcher's Smart Ones Bowl, Pasta Fagoli

Snack Foods
Ak-Mak 100% Whole-Wheat Crackers
Annie's Whole-Wheat Bunnies
Avo Classic Avocado Salsa Mix 'n' Dip
Back to Nature 100% Whole-Grain Baked Crackers
Back to Nature Roasted & Salted Soy Nuts
Barbara's Bakery Whole-Wheat Fig Bars
Blue Diamond Hazelnut Nut Thins Crackers
Certified Organic Just Fruit Munchies
Hain Pure Foods Wheatettes
Kashi TLC Original 7 Grain Crackers
Newman's Own Organic Unsalted Pretzel Rounds
Real Foods Rice Thins, Whole-Grain Rice Crackers
Ryvita Sesame Rye Whole-Grain Crispbread
Sahale Nut Blends
Seapoint Farm's Dry Roasted Edamame
Stretch Island Fruit Co. Fruit Leather

Juices and Beverages
8th Continent Complete Soy Milk
Harvest Bay Original Coconut Water
Heritage Foods Little Einstein Low-Fat Milk with DHA

Heritage Foods Organic Low-Fat Milk
Honest Tea Unsweetened, Just Black Tea
Lakewood Pure Cranberry Juice
Langer's All Pomegranate Juice
Millenium Synergy Tea
Natalie's Orchid Island Juice Company's Gourmet
    Pasteurized Orange Juice
Papa's Organic Grapefruit Juice
R.W. Knudsen Just Blueberry Juice
R.W. Knudsen Organic Tomato Juice
Silk Soy Milk with DHA
Simply Grapefruit 100% Juice
Stoneyfield Farm Organic Peach Smoothie
Sunsweet Prune Juice
Tropicana Pure and Natural Orange Juice
Tropicana Ruby-Red Grapefruit Juice
Welch's 100% Grape Juice

Sweets & Desserts
Bob's Red Mill Spice Apple Bran Muffin Mix
Brach's Wild & Fruity Sugar-Free Gummi Fruits
Breyers Double Churn Free Caramel Swirl
Breyers Nonfat Double Churn Free Cappuccino
    Chocolate Chunk
Ciao Bella Passion Fruit Sorbetto
Dole Strawberry Fruit 'n' Juice Bars
Dreyer's Fat-Free Frozen Yogurts
Dreyer's/Edy's Slow Churned Light Mint Chocolate Chip
Dreyer's Fruit Bars (Strawberry, Tangerine and Raspberry)
Friendly's Smooth Churned Light Vanilla or
    Light Forbidden Chocolate Ice Creams
Jolly Rancher Sugar-Free Candies
Jell-O Sugar-Free Raspberry
Jell-O Sugar-Free, Fat-Free Vanilla Pudding
Häagen-Dazs Fat-Free Raspberry Sorbet
Häagen-Dazs Fat-Free Sorbet and Yogurt
    (Raspberry and Vanilla bars)

Kashi TLC Oatmeal Raisin Flax Cookies
King Arthur Flour Cranberry-Orange Muffin Mix
Life Savers Mint O Green Sugar-Free
Martha's All-Natural Old-Fashioned Buttermilk
    Coffee Cake Mix
TCBY's Fat-Free yogurts
Tropicana Orange Juice Bar
Werther's Original Sugar-Free Caramels

INDEX